Hoopdance
Revolution

Hoopdance

Mindfulness in Motion

Revolution

FULL COLOR EDITION

Jan Camp

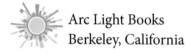
Arc Light Books
Berkeley, California

Hoopdance Revolution: Mindfulness in Motion

Every effort was made to credit photographs (page 231). If any has been overlooked, please alert the publisher: publisher@ArcLightBooks.com.

Arc Light Books are available at a discount when purchased in bulk.
Special editions or book excerpts can also be created to specification.
Contact: publisher@ArcLightBooks.com

Camp, Jan, 1946–
Hoopdance Revolution: Mindfulness in Motion: full color edition / Jan Camp
Includes references and Web links.
ISBN: 978-1-939353-01-6 (pbk. : alk. paper)
1. Hoop Exercises. 2. Hoop Dance. 3. Counterculture—United States—
History—21st century. I. Title.

Published by
Arc Light Books
Berkeley, California
www.ArcLightBooks.com

Cover, author, and flip photographs by Tom Weidlinger,
Arc Light Digital Media, www.ArcLightDigitalMedia.com

Cover and book design by Arc Light Books

Printed in the United States of America

INGRAM   10   9   8   7   6   5   4   3   2   1

To my partners in life, love, and art

*My whole life has been about waking up
and then waking up some more.*

—Sue Monk Kidd,
The Dance of the Dissident Daughter

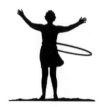

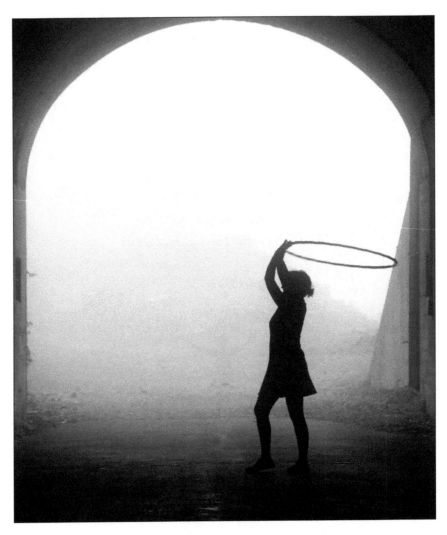

The author hoopdancing at the Marin Headlands in California

Contents

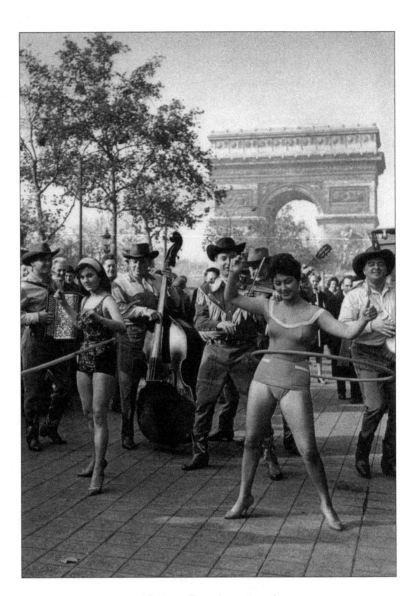

Vintage French postcard

Preface

My Call to the Hoop

During the 1950s, I spent hours playing with siblings and friends in the grassy backyard of my childhood home. For us life was a twenty-four-hour party, and we never wanted to stop running the length of the lawn—twirling, jumping, and singing songs from my older sister's 45s. "Whole lotta' shakin' goin' on . . . " and "I found my thrill on Blueberry Hill . . . " were lyrics we didn't fully understand and were not supposed to recite, but their rhythms captured the spirit of our play. When my father called us in for bed, we threw ourselves to the ground laughing or ran circles around him like cats refusing to be caught.

That rebellious energy continued to define my life until a condition in middle age threatened to stop me in my tracks. After years of physical therapy for chronic back pain I learned that muscle spasms and misaligned vertebrae were not the root cause of my trips to the emergency room. The severe turning of my head to the right and hips to the left was neurological in origin. A specialist called it *dystonia torticollis* and counseled, "Join a support group, and don't come back to my office because there is nothing I can do." Aging had superseded the party.

I explored everything from psychic healing to sound therapy and prescription drugs to prove the neurologist wrong. I relearned how to keep a normal posture and continued my work in fine art and graphic design. It was an improvement, but it was also difficult and disheartening. Then after buying myself a rocking chair with which to settle into old age, I received an e-mail about a hoopdance class at a yoga studio. Hula hooping with yoga? I had to see this. Convincing a friend that it might be fun to watch, even if we couldn't actually do it, we signed up.

In the class we were introduced to heavier, bigger hoops than we remembered from childhood. A typically lovely young instructor was our leader, and we held hoops throughout the warm-up exercises. Then as classmates struggled to coordinate limbs and core, we got rowdy and uncontrollable. We laughed—a lot!—reminiscent of our hula hooping as children.

Prior to the class I'd had little physical activity for several years. Suddenly, here was the hoop, bumping against my body, leading, resisting, 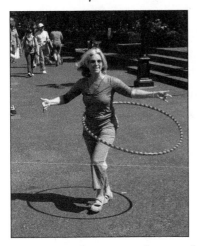 picking up momentum, and begging me to dance. It circumvented my neurological glitches by making me use muscles all over my body with irregular and therefore nonrepetitive movements. The hoop became a perfect biofeedback tool; it went clattering to the floor when erroneous messages were sent from my brain. At first there was nothing in my movements that you would call dancing. The jerky steps I took were more like Frankenstein's bride than the hooping I saw online, but I kept at it. I invited friends to the park, a grand extension of my own backyard. I brought hoops and music to share and couldn't help but invite strangers to join in as well. Hoopdance moved me quickly into an ecstatic mood. My heart chakra opened fully, and I understood viscerally what I had always held to be true: joy is the natural state of humankind. With persistent practice, I gradually regained equilibrium and established myself securely at a new level of health, awareness, and courage. Since aging is the party we're all going to, whether we want to or not, I suggest we bring hoops.

Introduction

A Brief History of Hooping

The hoopdance revolution officially started in the late 1990s with a handful of idealistic youth who followed the summer music festivals in the United States. Each took their colorful, oversized hoops back home to share with family and friends. From there the playful challenge of hoopdance grew into an international, intergenerational movement that invites us to feel good in our bodies and in our world.

Playing with hoops made from natural materials goes back to antiquity, but the advent of molded plastics made possible the manufacture and sale of over twenty million toy hoops during a few months. In 1958 the Hula Hoop caused one of the biggest fads ever documented by sociologists. At the same time, after thirteen years of postwar growth, with unemployment rising and auto sales falling, the United States was facing its first major recession since the Great Depression. In Europe and Canada many businesses and mining operations closed, causing exporting countries to suffer a decline in raw materials. Yet hula hooping took the world by storm. The Soviet Union denounced it as an example of empty American culture, and Japan banned the hoop to prevent immodest behavior.

After its initial success, the plastic hoop became a toy-box staple that was promoted now and again, especially in times of trouble. It resurfaced during the Vietnam War, and in 1968 the Wham-O Manufacturing Company, creator of the Hula Hoop, began collaborating with the National Parks & Recreation Network. In competitions later named the World Hula Hoop Championships, competitors were judged on the performance of specific maneuvers; and freestyle routines set to music established a root of the contemporary hoopdance movement.

Then hooping seemed to disappear from popular consciousness once again, only to return in the early 1980s with another recession. Barry Shapiro, Wham-O's executive vice president and general manager in 1982, said, "Wham-O has always felt that when the world is in kind of a messy way, and people are unhappy, something like the hoop lets them just forget everything while they go spinning around."[1]

The World Hula Hoop Championships grew from five hundred host cities in 1968 to over two thousand in the 1980s, with two million participants. National competitions were exported and staged in Germany, the Netherlands, and the United Kingdom. Then in 1987 Mat Plendl's performance on national television transformed the phenomenon of child's play into adult pop culture. As hooping emerged in the following decade, distinct styles developed and spread.

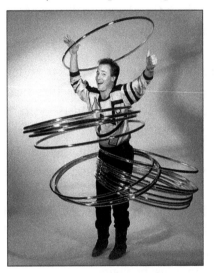 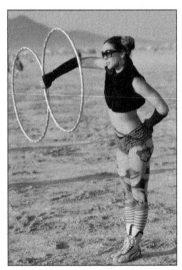

Mat Plendl, 1987   Spiral, 2010

By 1991 Paul Blair was using a hoop to dance at music concerts in Washington State. Later he supplied larger hoops to the String Cheese Incident band in Colorado. The band took hoops to music festivals and threw them from the stage to get people moving. Betty Shurin and Anah Reichenbach were in the audience in 1997, and hoopdancing changed their lives. Betty holds world records and hoops while snowboarding. Anah introduced hoopdance to the Los Angeles nightclub and rave scene and went on the road as "Hoopalicious" to sell her handmade hoops.

In 2001, Vivian Hancock (aka Spiral) took her String Cheese Incident hoop back to the little town of Carrboro, North Carolina. Together with Julia Hartsell and Jonathan Baxter, she formed a community that others continue to travel to for hooping camaraderie. At the same time members of Groovehoops were meeting in New York's Central Park, because as Stefan Pildes says, "After 9/11 it was important to be with friends and play." All across the country, people were rediscovering hula hooping in a new form, with bigger hoops for dancing, performing, and healing. Michele Clark, an original member of Groovehoops, says, "The magic of hoopdance is in the physical process of creative learning. Neural pathways are reconstructed when you spontaneously let each thing you do lead to the next. It changes you."

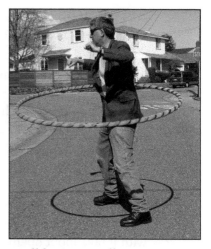

My husband, Tom Weidlinger, is a documentary filmmaker who often spends more time at his desk writing, researching, and editing than he does moving about on location. He started hooping to relieve his sciatica pain, and because he is six foot six, I made him a five-foot diameter hoop with one-inch tubing. Going beyond waist hooping, he exercises shoulders, wrists, and spine as well as his lower back. Tom and I both work from home and on most days we add a hoop session to our coffee break, in the street in front of our home.

In Chicago Heather Crosby hoopdanced in small bars, as well as in front of sixty thousand spectators at Soldier Field, but she was uncomfortable with being in the spotlight. She established Hooper Power to teach classes and workshops as a more personal way of sharing her connection to the hoop with others.

Hooping.org columnist Lara Eastburn felt completely involved in the hooping community from behind her computer screen but she worried about going to her first in-person hoop gathering, "What if I'm the odd one out in groups of old friends?" When she got there, familiar online avatars sprang to life as real and welcoming faces. Her Hooping Family Tree Project charted hoopdance worldwide, documenting its genealogy from inception to 2012. For instance, my hoopdance lineage goes like this: Dizzy Hips → String Cheese Incident → Hoopalicious → HoopGirl → Rosie Lila → Jan Camp. (See the full project results at www.hoopdancebook.com/family-tree.)

How to Use the Book

Hoopdance Revolution tells the story of a cultural movement while providing tips and practical examples for applying hoopdance philosophy. You can follow a tenet of sports psychology to let creative visualization support your hoopdance training. As you read, flip the bottom corner of the book pages, or watch and listen to optional Web links (referenced V and M in the text), just imagine that you are practicing with the hoop.

Lists of links at the end of each chapter are accompanied by Quick Response (QR) codes, like the one below for the book's website. Mobile devices such as your phone or tablet can read the QR, with a QR reader app installed. Each QR points to the website page containing media samples for the chapter in which it appears.

The book's website hosts its own 30-second video clips and the book's trailer, as well as links to source videos and other hoopdance-related websites at www.HoopDanceBook.com.

Part Descriptions

Part I: Into the Circle. The hoop is a simple circle, yet people who connect with it talk about opening their lives to synchronicity, deep healing, and flow. Read stories about the physical and emotional benefits of hooping for children and adults. Learn to make a hoop, warm up, waist hoop, and practice playful exercises.

Part II: The Revolution. All you need to join the revolution, no matter what your age or size, is a hoop that's right for you and a generous portion of passion, persistence, and letting go. Join the author as she meets individuals who used hoops distributed by the String Cheese Incident band to spread the practice of hoopdance. Find out how you can connect on the Internet, why people join the movement, and where they gather.

Part III: Hoopdance. Hoop performers bridge two styles: trick-oriented circus arts and contemporary-flow hoopdance. See how the movement generates a myriad of combinations of clothing, tools, and sound; shares technique with juggling, yoga, and martial arts; and how it is used for charity toward others and for personal spiritual growth.

List of Key Profiles

Listed by first name, with the page number of the main profile.

Note

1. "Dividends: Grandson of Hula Hoop," *Time,* March 15, 1982.

PART I

Into the Circle

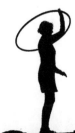

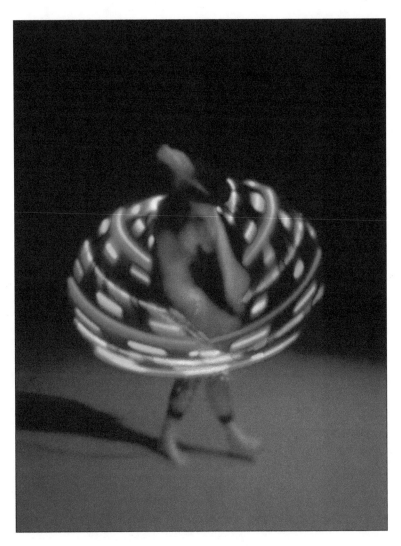

Emma Kerr at the LED Hoopers' Ball

ONE

Synchronicity and Flow

You can only have good thoughts while hooping.
Anything negative just shoots out from the circle and fun comes in.
—Kevin O'Keeffe, World Hoop Day organizer

The sensation of whirling like a dervish as a young woman, my skirts billowing with centrifugal force, returned to me during my very first hoopdance class. Along with seven other students, I gave the instructor my full attention even though I was unsure that I would be able to manage a large hoop. When she demonstrated the graceful flow of hoopdancing, however, there was no turning back: I was going to do *that*. Before long we were swinging hoops wildly and dropping them freely. By the middle of the class I was gaining control of my hoop; by the end, I was committed to the practice. It was fun, aerobic, and social.

At home I started practicing for just one minute a day in my driveway with a high fence to shield my awkward attempts. On rainy days I pushed aside the furniture and hooped in my living room to the music of Buena Vista Social Club, Janis Ian, or Yo-Yo Ma, depending on my mood. As I progressed I wanted company; I wanted laughter and inspiration as well as the dance. I made hoops for all my friends from instructions I found on the Internet, and moved from the safety of my driveway to the 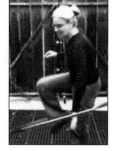 park around the corner. "I could never do it" became my cue to help others reach that moment of elation when, for the first time, the hoop orbits the body and stays up, even if only for a revolution or two.

3

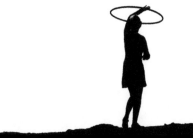

In those first few months I rapidly dropped twelve pounds, began to dress in clothes that hugged my body, and explored types of music that I had never thought to listen to before. I loved everyone and everything. It was exciting, wonderful, and a little disconcerting. For a time I felt out of control. My body was changing fast, and my moods often elevated to inappropriate heights. As frightening as it sometimes felt, I didn't give up the hoop. Instead I began to use hoopdance for balance, integrating it into my spiritual practice as a way to calm my mind and celebrate life.

Before long I wanted to know everything about this phenomenal tool that was reconstructing my entire outlook: Where did hoopdance come from? Who else is doing it? Does everyone undergo profound transformation? The few books and many websites I found sparked my curiosity further. In the end by meeting and playing with hoopdancers, and interviewing them about their experiences, I came to understand the significance of the hoop as a catalyst for energetic change.

Hoop Roots

Hoops made from grapevines were used in ancient Egypt as early as 1000 B.C.E., and the Greek physician Hippocrates, the father of Western medicine, prescribed hoop rolling to exercise a weak back. In fourteenth-century England, adults as well as children enjoyed hooping around the

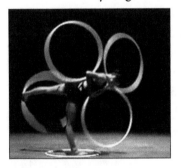

waist. Later sailors on Pacific Island voyages connected waist hooping with hula dancing and coined the term "hula hooping." In the nineteenth century, hoop rolling and hoop juggling came to the variety stage. Hoop rolling has been popular on U.S. college campuses since the late 1890s, and in 2012 the "Hoopie Award," honoring the year's best video of hoopdancing, went to a hoop juggler.[1] V

Hoop rolling is a game in which a hoop is trundled with a stick to keep it upright or to do tricks.

Hula dancing is native to Hawaii,
dramatizing oral history through song and movement.

Synchronicity

In 2009 I was a hoopdance novice, teaching the moves I learned at introductory classes in California to my friends in the park. My sister Chris, an occupational therapist on the other side of the country, had seen me hoopdance and asked me to help her buy her first hoop. She wanted to try it but was overwhelmed looking for the right tubing in hardware stores. I suggested she look for a teacher instead, because most instructors make and sell hoops in a variety of sizes, weights, and colorful patterns. Not only could she try out several before buying one, but taking a series of classes would be a great way for her to get started. She would make new friends over time while learning how to dance and execute moves.

Before my flight back east, a fellow student brought a light-emitting diode (LED) hoop to a class I took in Berkeley. I had only seen LED hoops on the Internet, and he had purchased his online from a company called Hooping Harmony.

Unlike the diagonally patterned hoops sold in most of my classes, this one was made of white polymer tubing sectioned off with vertical stripes of tape. Before it was activated it looked like the hoops used by American Indian hoop dancers. But when the LED hoop lit up, its bare sections glowed with color from within while its owner danced like a swirling aurora borealis. We all got to try it. When it was my turn, I twirled the luminous color up and down my body as if I were inside a star.

Then I flew back east to meet Chris in the little town of Easthampton, Massachusetts before our annual family picnic, and I brought my collapsible travel hoop. It folds into a figure eight and then in half again as two small circles that fit easily through security screening machines. Although it draws a bit of attention, I don't mind coming up with amusing answers to questions like, "What do you do with those little circus hoops?"

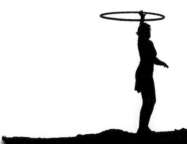

Before the picnic, Chris and I went up the road to Greenfield to check out the teacher she had found, and to shop for her hoop. I had lived in Greenfield as a hippie mom in the 1970s, which was then known as a place of spiritual healing. Once we got off the new highway and into the neighborhood, it didn't seem that much had changed. The air shimmered with possibility as we parked in front of a large, brick, gambrel-roofed home on a tree-lined street and followed our directions to the back entrance. Halfway up a steep stairway, hoops were hanging on the wall. More were stacked on the next landing. We were definitely in the right place.

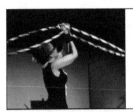

LED hoops are used by performance and circus artist Alley 'Oop.[2] [V]

Hooping Harmony

When we reached the top landing, Chris and I were greeted by Ariana Shelton and her business partner, Laura Marie, two lovely women. Once inside, I caught sight of a stash of LED hoops exactly like the one I'd seen in class. We had arrived at the home base of Hooping Harmony—a mother-and-daughter cottage industry that does an impressive amount of hoop production, counseling, and teaching with a small crew of volunteers.

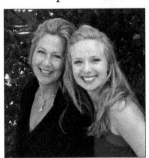

The primary work of Hooping Harmony is holistic fitness: the well-being of body, mind, and spirit. Together Ariana and Laura focus their understanding of human nature and how things work, on creating systemic change in the world. Adding one hoopdancer at a time to a groundswell shift, they shape their classes and events to assure each student some level of comfort and success by providing a large selection of hoops, plenty of space, and enough trained helpers for assistance. Chris signed up for a Hooping Harmony YMCA class on the spot.

Wherever Ariana and Laura go with hoops they are treated like celebrities. A neighbor offers to store overflow inventory. An elderly woman asks what they've got there, and Laura gives an impromptu demonstration.

Kids follow them like the Pied Piper. Laura finds that in most people's minds, the hoop means freedom, childhood, and fun. "I've watched people step into the hoop with a negative outlook and seen them begin to lighten. Some part of them opens up. With practice they begin to feel better about themselves and to actually enjoy each other more. It's beautiful to watch."

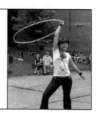

When Laura hoopdances at the park, she has a willing audience.[3] [V]

Laura discovered hooping in 2006 the way many people do, in the park where she had gone to meet a friend. "There were some big hoops just lying around. Neither of us had been able to hoop as children, but we thought, 'What the heck,' and tried." Laura overcame her childhood failure in a transcendent moment. It left her with such an elated feeling that she went home and told Ariana, "Mom, you've got to check this out."

Ariana realized with her first attempt that she could use hooping in her practice as a holistic health consultant. "When Laura and I started, no one talked about health benefits. Most of the hoopdancers we found online were focused on performance. For them it was about feeling sensual and getting sexy but we knew it could be used for fitness. For two days, information about the potential of the hooping movement poured through me." Working as an intuitive healer and life coach in a conservative part of the country, the hoop allows Ariana to reach those people who are skeptical of any "healing" that does not take place in a doctor's office. With it she helps them hoop past their wariness, to achieve new levels of well-being.

Though she was born in 1958, the year that toy hoops caused the biggest surge of interest in hooping history, Ariana started hooping later in life. And she was the only serious hooper of her age that she and Laura knew about at the time. "We were up here by ourselves working it out, but we knew it was going to be big. This remake from the 1950s was growing, and it was not going to go away." Her age was to their advantage when

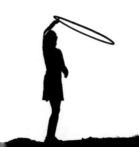

she and her daughter decided to develop a line of hoops. The needs of Ariana's mature body suggested they create something gentler than the heavy hoops with which they had started. They made smaller and lighter ones to avoid damage to arms and hands, and larger, medium-weight ones to make learning new moves easier. But Ariana still likes the feeling and rhythm of a larger hoop around her waist.

Laura has been making things her whole life so figuring out how to make hoops was a challenge she took to naturally. "We just started buying stuff. Tubing wasn't easy to find. We went into some places where I thought, 'Whoa, women probably never come in here.'" Baffled men asked them, "You want what—for what?" It was a learning curve. Some of the tapes they tried gave Laura a rash and had an odor that made Ariana feel sick. Eventually they found nontoxic tapes to use on their hoops.

Deep Healing

By 2007 Ariana and Laura had immersed themselves in the business of hoopdance. They entered their yes year, responding eagerly to requests to work with hospital psychiatric units, infectious disease units, and groups for children, survivors of abuse, and teenage boys at-risk. They asked of themselves, "Can hooping make a difference?" and found that in many circumstances it helped individuals feel better about themselves. Ariana made sure that every one of her therapy clients went home with a hoop.

A woman I'll call Madeline came from Boston for counseling. She is as tall as Ariana, but she walked hunched over and quickly sat down on a low couch so that she seemed small and meek. At the end of her first session she bought a hoop in shades of blue and silver. Laura showed her how to use it, and Madeline asked if Hooping Harmony would donate a demonstration to the nonprofit organization she directed. Laura and Ariana agreed to meet her there after three months.

Back in Boston Madeline went out onto her balcony every morning to waist hoop for ten minutes in one direction and ten minutes in the other. When Ariana and Laura showed up for their demonstration seminar, a person they hardly recognized bounded out to meet them. Laura asked her mother, "Who's that?" and Ariana said, "Oh my goodness, that's my client!" Madeline told them she had lost thirty-five pounds and had started dating. Hooping had so positively altered her life that she had integrated hoop breaks into the workday. Hooping made her entire staff happier and more engaged in their work.

For others, the space inside the hoop's tangible boundary created a comforting sense of safety. A couple I'll call David and Anita came to Ariana together. There was abundant love between them, but they had developed a pattern of intense bickering whenever one person's needs conflicted with those of the other.

Ariana didn't tell them to stop fighting. Instead she suggested that the couple get into their hoops at the first sign of trouble and keep them circling their waists as they argued. David and Anita agreed, and within six weeks they had broken their disruptive habit. Keeping the hoop going diverted attention from their disagreement and allowed the underlying trust they had in each other to resurface and overshadow feelings of neediness. David and Anita learned over time that speaking to each other from a place of love is more productive than being right.

Flow and the Physical Core

In her hoopdance classes Ariana continually brought students back to the balance and rhythm of basic fitness. Early on she noticed that a group of her older students, in their fifties and sixties, were becoming dynamic hoopdancers. By paying attention to their posture they were gaining freedom of expression. In contrast the movement of youngsters, focusing on the number of tricks they could master, appeared choppy and disconnected. This raised the questions: Once you've got your moves, how will you use them? How will you find your flow?

Physical elegance and the ability to lose yourself in the beauty of movement come in large part from a strong and flexible core, the muscles from your rib cage to pelvic floor, including the psoas and abdominals that stabilize the spine. When I started hooping, I realized that I had lost touch with the deeper muscles of my core. Luckily I found yoga classes in a physical therapy clinic that helped me reconnect. Pairing yoga with hoopdance helps me prevent injury, and I learn about my body with mindfulness from two perspectives. In hoopdance I interact with the hoop through

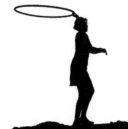

resistance and yielding on the fly. In yoga I focus energy on resistance and yielding within my tissue and bones, slowly and methodically.

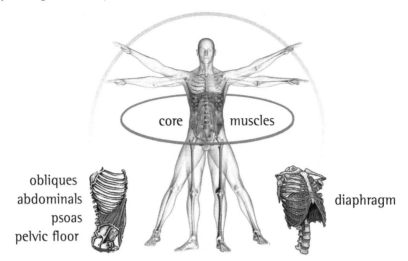

obliques
abdominals
psoas
pelvic floor
diaphragm

To flow in hoopdance requires muscle memory, physical knowledge gained by the body through practice over time. It helps us to smooth out the tricks we learn by drawing on patterns stored in our muscles, rather than thinking about what we will do next. We manipulate the hoop, creating tempo and phrasing. Information then comes back from the hoop to our nerve endings. Like tiny hands at the ready, they activate the subtle movements that keep the hoop aloft. The more I dance, the better I become at knowing when my body, hoop, and spirit are in sync, and when they are out of balance. Learning to use core muscles as the hub of my action, allows my arms and legs to move both powerfully and gracefully.

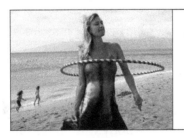

In California Kaye Anderson leads classes in hoopdance. She says: "When body and hoop become one in movement, that's flow."

Because Laura Marie had been dancing since she was three, she and Ariana understood the importance of core conditioning within the broader scope of biomechanics, the study of movement within our biological structure. When Laura started hoopdancing, she noticed, in the few performance videos available online, that people were not paying much attention to how they positioned their feet and hips. She knew that could lead to problems with ankles and knees. By "micro-moving" over and over again, Laura broke down each move until she and Ariana understood its biomechanics precisely enough to teach it safely to their students.

Start by thinking of the body as three interdependent sections:

- The upper body, from the top of the head to the ribs, including the arms.
- The midsection or "core," from the top of the diaphragm to the pelvic floor.
- The lower body, from the hips through the legs to the soles of the feet.

Anah Reichenbach is a master of flow. She describes the technique of shoulder hooping as allowing the hoop to flow across the body from front to back as you gently push with your shoulders from side to side. Her bare midriff makes the interdependence of core muscles visible when she teaches this technique.[4] 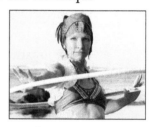 (See the end of chapter 5 for shoulder hooping.)

Anah choreographs only the beginning and end of her performance, leaving the middle open to flow in the moment. "Once, watching a video of myself," she told me, "I was surprised to see that I had hoopdanced backwards down a few stairs while turning onto the main stage. I wasn't familiar with that stage, but I was able to navigate the space because I was in the flow of my dance." To get to that state of flow, Anah has to work out and practice. It takes a lot of repetition and persistence to have the physical and emotional proficiency to let go in unfamiliar territory.

A Contagious State of Mind

Mihaly Csikszentmihalyi is the chief architect of creative flow psychology and the author of *Flow: The Psychology of Optimal Experience.* I met him in 1993 at a seminar for broadcast journalists at the University of Chicago.

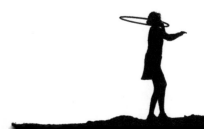

He described flow as the state we enter when we are fully absorbed in what we are doing and our sense of time is given over to feelings of great satisfaction. "Every action, movement, and thought follows inevitably from the previous one. Your whole being is involved, and you use your skills to the utmost."

Richard Hartnell is a contact juggler who draws on Csikszentmihalyi's studies. In his video, *The Meaning of Flow,* Hartnell posits that, consciously 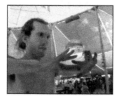 or not, all human beings seek out the mind state of egolessness that we find in deep concentration. He narrates, "When the doer is completely absorbed by the task at hand, there is incredible ease, time slows down, and space expands to create moments of complete lucidity."[5] V

Connecting core fitness with your own style and an optimal state of mind leads to flow. When you invest in flow, change happens—in you, in the energetic space around you, and in your relationship to others.

Before my sister Chris could begin her hoopdance changes, she had to buy a hoop. There were many to choose from at Hooping Harmony, and she tried several before she bought the one in earth tones that felt right to her. Laura Marie sold us blank hoops as well. She connected bare black tubing into circles that we could decorate with tape I brought from home.

I learned about adding tape to hoops at Hooping.org, an online magazine published and edited by Philo Hagen. According to legend Philo uploaded stories from the taxi he drove in San Francisco, but he says that even though he drove a cab there before moving to Los Angeles, he always uses the computer on his desk to edit the website. He recalls that even as a cab driver he experienced flow: "I would drop someone off and someone else might be there waiting for a ride. It's the stream of 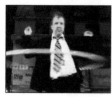 life. Taxi driving taught me about being present, in the right place at the right time." Philo's video *Gotta Hoop* gets to the bare essentials of hoopdance flow. It contrasts the boredom of working in a cubicle with the allure of hooping and the thrill of daring to try something new.[6] V

Flow can be contagious. Studies show that brain waves emanating from a person in a state of flow not only affect him or her but also influence the brain waves of others in close proximity. Hoopdancer Michele Clark

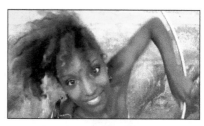

experienced both synchronicity and flow when the band Phish gave a reunion concert at Madison Square Garden on New Year's Eve 2002. She and her friends had spent the day dressing in elaborate costumes and hairdos even though they didn't have advance tickets.

With over thirty thousand people trying to get into the show, of course the box office was sold out, and thousands of people were standing on the corner of Thirty-fourth Street and Eighth Avenue when Michele started hooping to the music in her head. "I was getting energy from the crowd that had condensed around me, and my peers were getting to see me shine with the hoop. It was a moment of total ecstatic sensation." She was putting energy out and getting it back. She was in flow.

Then as Michele and her friends were deciding what to do next, Phish guitarist Trey Anastasio emerged from the crowd and gave them each a ticket. Michele says, "It was like moving from one high to an even higher high. It was epic. I loved that hooping was my new life. I had never jumped up and down or screamed in public, but in that moment I understood what people at Michael Jackson concerts felt when they fainted and pulled out their hair." Michele and her friends' tickets were for seats next to other friends. "We all sat together—that's synchronicity."

Family and Friends

Chris and I showed up at our family's picnic with five hoops. Forty-five relatives were happy to watch us hoopdancing, and even though it rained off and on, some of our siblings and cousins joined in. My cousin Frankie's granddaughter, nine-year-old Kayla, was particularly good at it. Her pace was steady, her timing impeccable. Unlike the haphazard fun most of us were having, she pushed the hoop just where and when it was needed, completely focused, walking and hooping through the noisy, laughing crowd.

Kayla had been using her own small hoop at home. Her mom told me, "Before Kayla started hooping she was uncoordinated and had a hard time

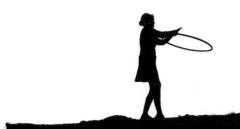

concentrating. She didn't like to interact with people." At the picnic Kayla was eager for my suggestions. I showed her how to change her hoop's

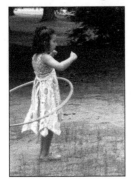

direction and to rotate the hoop around her hand. When her core muscles tired, she practiced hand moves. She checked in with me to show her progress using a toy hoop off body to move with her hands, and around her waist she twirled a hoop clockwise and counterclockwise that was at least as wide as she was tall.

It is always a nostalgic pleasure to be in the circle of loving relatives, but sharing a new activity with my extended family made our 2009 picnic exceptional.

Is Hoopdance for You?

When you have the unique experience of hoopdance in common with people you love, it deepens relationships. But not everyone who tries hoop-

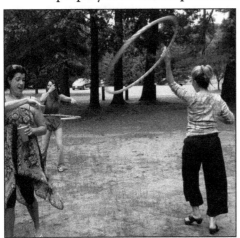

ing will stay with it, even if they love it at first. What will keep you engaged when others leave it behind? Community is a crucial ingredient for most people. Sharing hoopdance in classes or for performance and particularly at jams, where everyone is teacher, performer, and student at once, supports an ongoing practice. If you already have a creative community and a workout routine that is keeping you fit, you may not get the hoopdance bug. Or you may learn to

hoop, practice for a while, and then stop doing it because of a physical complaint, self-consciousness, or limited time. Most of all you have to love movement, even if that means dropping the hoop. The sound a hoop makes when it falls lets you know where your edge is, and listening to it builds an interaction that lasts.

Hoopdance often highlights problems that require our attention. To work through stumbling blocks, start slowly, especially if you are out of shape or overly stressed. Try using different hoops to find one that engages you in a feeling of pleasure, and adjust your posture when you feel yourself slumping into repetition, discomfort, or strain. Be aware of your attitude, breathe gently into areas of difficulty, sending energy there, and remain open to the possibility of breakthrough. Transformation that sneaks into our lives as something light and playful can often bring the deepest and most lasting benefits.

Changes that are made slowly give the body time to grow into its new shape. If you hoop regularly, for just a minute a day, it might lead to a song per session. From there you can increase incrementally until you are getting the workout you need. If you can't find a solid block of time, practice for shorter periods more often. If you allow yourself to get lost in the movement of your hoop, you will naturally find what works for you.

Chapter One Links

www.HoopDanceBook.com/chapter1

1. *Raw: Ring-o-graphy.* Jan. 8, 2012.

2. *Alley'Oop Hoop with Wonderbolt Circus.* Sep. 30, 2009.

3. *Laura Marie of Hooping Harmony at Pulaski Park.* Jul. 26, 2009.

4. *Hoop Dance Tutorial: Shoulder Hooping Techniques with Anah Reichenbach.* Jan. 1, 2012.

5. *Flowtoys—"The Meaning of Flow" (Richard Hartnell).* Dec. 9, 2010.

6. *Hooping.org Presents: Gotta Hoop.* Nov. 8, 2010.

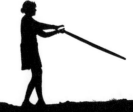

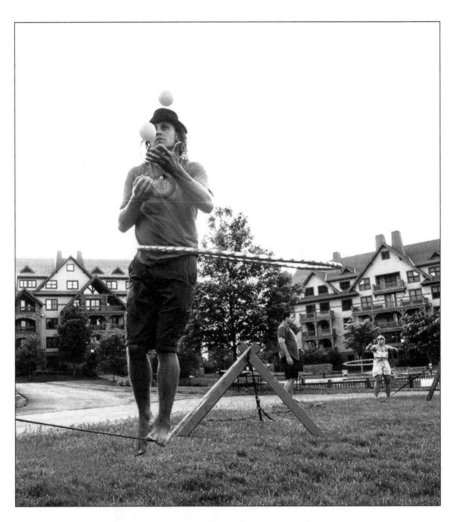
Sam Salwei hooping and juggling on a slackline

TWO

The Basics

I felt giddy and euphoric . . . like I had finally cleared
some ancient gym-class hurdle I'd forgotten was there.

—Sean Cole, journalist (hooping for the first time)

Editor of Hooping.org, Philo Hagen, was frequently asked to post the size
and weight of hoops used in each of the "Tutorial of the Week" videos he
posted. He recounts, "Often readers want to know exactly what size hoop
is necessary for each specific trick. The answer doesn't matter because
everyone's body is physically different. The hoop that rocks one person's
world may be too big or too small for someone else doing the same thing."

Size Matters

A general rule suggests that hoops should be forty-two inches in diameter
or smaller, but for some, range of motion, physical ability, and body size
might call for a hoop that stands fifty inches or more. If a hoop is too small
for you, or too light, it will be hard to control; if it's too heavy, your body
might not be able to communicate with its rhythm, or you may quickly
become tired. Start with a hoop that complements your size and shape,
whatever they might be.

Keep several hoops on hand. At minimum, one that is a
perfect size for your present comfort zone, a smaller
one to use off-body or to challenge your skills,
and a larger one for trying new techniques.

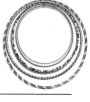

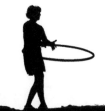

A large hoop makes getting started and learning new tricks easier because it rotates more slowly. A smaller hoop spins faster for more challenge, fancy dancing, and hand moves. The hoopdance trend for developing complex movements that require smaller hoops was a natural direction because staying in flow requires that challenge and skill levels are matched in such a way that new awareness can emerge. Paradoxically once you master smaller hoops you may eventually be challenged by larger ones.

Large diameter, heavier material = slower = easier.
Smaller diameter, lighter material = faster = more difficult.

Dancing with hoops of different sizes not only varies your experience but it affects the aesthetic. Teacher/performer Rosie Lila (Miss Rosie) is a long-limbed woman. After a demonstration in which she used a thirty-five-inch hoop, a friend suggested that the size was limiting her physical expression. Switching to a thirty-six-inch diameter was an elegant solution. It gave Miss Rosie a little extra time to make more graceful transitions.

Names Matter

Hoopers coming into the movement, where online presence is a driving force, often choose alter-ego names to embrace new personas. Early performers and teachers jump-started the tradition of hoop names by creating business and stage names.

According to legend, hooper names got started when Anah Reichenbach (Hoopalicious) asked her performance partners in Los Angeles to choose stage names.

Naming events are common at raves for anonymity, and alter egos are used for Internet social networking.

Playa or Burner nicknames are chosen by some and earned by others to differentiate a particular Michelle, Patrick, or Vivian from others at Burning Man, the annual art festival and temporary community, on a playa in Nevada.

At the Burning Man festival (the Burn), a performance artist called BunnyMan spins hoops that are six to eight feet and more in diameter. His moniker is typical of pseudonyms in the hoopdance community. On the playa BunnyMan wears a white suit, often with a black armband. "I use black hoops as an anti-war statement. The metaphor is about going around in circles and not really 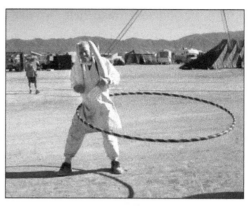 accomplishing anything, and I have jokes to go along with each trick. This makes some people, who might otherwise be having a great time hooping, drop the hoop and leave because they don't want to protest a war."

BunnyMan was introduced to hooping by circus performers who practiced in the building he managed, a warehouse of artists' studios on Marigny Street in the Faubourg Marigny section of New Orleans. The area abuts the Bywater Ninth Ward, a district that was devastated by Hurricane Katrina. There was a heavy National Guard presence in the Marigny Rectangle after the storm. BunnyMan remembers a guardsman ordering him to get out of the street with his hoop. He told the officer, "It's an eight-foot hoop! It isn't going to fit on the sidewalk." The guardsman stood firm even though there was no traffic.

In 2009 I visited BunnyMan, and we went to a Day of the Dead parade. Waiting for it to begin, we watched crusty punks (young people noted for street entertaining and homelessness) gather into an amiable crowd. Judging from the number of cell phones in use and the pungent aromas mingling in the fall air, the group also included a few upper crusties and a number of soap dodgers (those who have means of support and others opposed to bathing). Dogs barked and people chatted. A young woman shared *miel* wine from a mason jar. We sat on the edge of a concrete foundation where revelers took turns using BunnyMan's massive hoops. "They love to use my hoops down here in New Orleans," he said, "but they don't

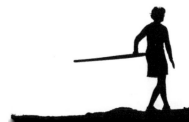

go out and make their own like in other places. Hooping just hasn't caught on here in that way."

I thought that the Big Easy might not need hooping because it already has many reasons to dress up, move, and party, but at the House of Blues later that night, an LED hoop duet rocked the house. Stefan Pildes, from Groovehoops in New York, performed with DJ Brent Van Dyke to the band Billi Shakes and the Phakespeare Orchestra. It was 1920s-style cabaret, with sassy hip-hop, digital effects, and hoopdancing.

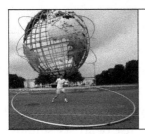

In 2010 Ashrita Furman successfully twirled a hoop that was 198.7 inches in diameter. Achieving Guinness World Records is his wacky spiritual practice.[1] V

Crafting the Hoop

Historically hoops have been made of vines, reeds, metal bands, and bent wood. When I started hoopdancing, everyone I asked thought that hula hooping was invented in 1958 when the toy company Wham-O sold a record number of lightweight plastic hoops. In fact, Australian school-children were hooping in physical education classes with wooden hoops before plastic hoops became a twentieth-century phenomenon. You can probably still buy a plastic hoop at your local toy store, larger dance hoops are sold over the Internet and at classes and workshops, and you can make your own. Regardless of how your hoop is made, its perfection is in how you relate to it and how it performs for you. Adults generally need something more substantial than a toy hoop, and kids love bigger hoops too. For most of us a good rule of thumb is to start with a hoop that, when stood on edge in front of you, will reach somewhere between your naval and breastbone. (Instructions for making an irrigation-tubing hoop are at the end of this chapter.)

Eco-Friendlier Material

Even though PVC products do not emit toxins in their solid form, the manufacturing and disposal of plastics are problematic for the environment.

Eco Faeries in New Zealand suggest that we reuse discarded piping that is on its way to the landfill. Patrick Deluz of PsiHoops in California says, "I would like to find a material that is biodegradable yet translucent. I made a hoop with woven twigs, and I tried to grow bamboo hoops, but the results were less than immaculate."

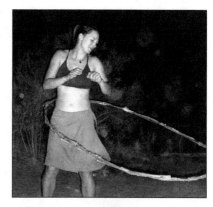

Irrigation tubing and tape to decorate our hoops are made from petroleum. In an oil-scarce future what will our hoops be made of? I was impressed when I saw the hoop that physical therapist Lori Hoffmann and her friend Portland firefighter Audrey Tolefson made during a two-week rafting trip on the Colorado River. On a layover day they wanted to hoop, so they used materials they had at hand: tamarisk branches and duct tape.

I decided to try my hand at going back to nature. Where I live in Berkeley there is plenty of bamboo, so first I harvested some from a friend's yard. I soaked it in water for several days, but it was still too rigid to bend. Then I got lucky when it was time to trim my thornless rose. The Lady Banks Yellow Rose puts out long shoots that are beautifully pliable. I cut a couple of the longest branches and doubled up the thin ends, tying them onto one of my sturdiest conventional hoops to dry into a circle. I freed the rose-vine hoop from its support after a couple of weeks and tied colorful strips of fabric to it. It was seasoned enough for a test, and I hoopdanced to the album *Book of Roses* by Andreas Vollenweider. With the bonus of being ecologically virtuous, the rose hoop is one of my favorite toys.

In 2012 HoopRevolution.com created the EcoHoop. It is a high quality, high performance, portable hoop that is recycled and recyclable. Good for us all and good for the earth, it could help to reduce billions of pounds of plastic waste. If you like making things, experiment with whatever natural materials you can find to come up with your own perfect hoop solution, and to spare our environment some toxins.

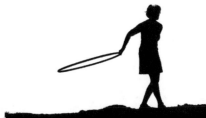

Warm Up, Hoopdance, and Stretch

Warming up your muscles is an important step before you use your hoop. Athletes—yes, hoopers are athletes—achieve maximum potential in any field by first bringing the body to attention, and connecting with a deep internal place during warm-up. Warming up to music helps engage the mind, body, and spirit in the mood of the practice, workout, or performance to come.

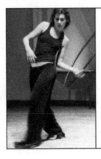

Hoopdancer Brecken Rivara says: "When you are warming up, don't stretch your muscles— make lines with your body." She refers to dancers' body lines, created by the movement and extension of limbs in space.

Take it easy warming up and save intense stretching for after hooping, when contracted muscles may need increased circulation to reduce lactic acid and restore flexibility and comfort. Ten minutes of movement before you start hooping and ten for stretching after will usually do the job. During a good warm-up, as energy moves through every part of your body, natural lubrication becomes more fluid, coating and protecting joints to improve mobility and prevent injury.

Start by letting your mind drop into your body. Feel the rhythm of the silence or the tempo of the music. Move gently and freely to awaken muscles. As you walk the space with or without the hoop, feel the energy in your feet connect you to the earth. Notice the expanse above your head. Survey your surroundings. Engage the triangular surface of your feet from the oval pads behind your toes to the circles of your heels. Prance, alternating between pointed and flexed feet to bring energy into your ankles and lower legs. Stretch the sides of your body by reaching in every direction while keeping shoulders securely in their sockets. And let your nose lead your head and neck to make little figure eights in the air. Later your hoop can guide your whole body in making a powerful figure-eight motion. When you feel ready, amp up the music and get into your hoop.

While warming up:

- Notice how the components of your core move with and opposite to each other.
- Mirror your movement in one direction with the same movement in the opposite direction.
- Get used to moving the upper, core, and lower sections of the body interdependently.

(Exercises for warming up, basic waist hooping, and stretching are included at the end of the chapter.)

Tips for Learning to Hoop

If you are new to hooping, avoid using your body as a single unit like a paddle. Taking a rigid stance might help to keep the hoop up longer, but it will make dancing more difficult and ultimately cause strain. Instead, keep your posture loose and responsive, even if it means dropping the hoop more often. That's half the fun.

Reversing direction improves balance and mental acuity by engaging both sides of the body and the brain. In North Carolina, hoop teacher Carolyn Mabry (Caroleeena) uses reversals to engage her "energy fields," the electromagnetic system that extends outward from her body. In hoopdance practice she alternates swirling things away from herself and drawing things into her circle.[2]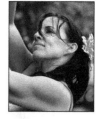

Start practicing in both directions right away, clockwise (to the right) and counterclockwise (to the left). You will notice that one direction is easier than the other. When you master coordination in your easier, or dominant, direction, the body stores information in your muscles to help you gain proficiency in the more difficult, opposite direction.

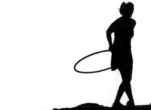

Betty Shurin (Betty Hoops) advises that you hold the hoop level because a wobbly hoop will not spin.

Christabel Zamor's fitness program HoopGirl uses the term "pump" to describe the front-to-back motion.

Jonathan Livingston Baxter founded the HoopPath and uses a blindfold to better understand the body-hoop connection.

Closing your eyes can help you feel the hoop's motion and timing more clearly while learning to keep it on a horizontal plane around your waist equally well in both directions. Alternate with simple hand rotations to develop intuitive control and gain flexible strength. Moving on to hoopdance, you will add expressive arm movements, footwork, and directed gaze, as you invent tricks or try moves you see in videos and learn at classes. Once you are hoopdancing on your own, consider doing it with a partner to heighten challenge, fun, and trust.

Duet hooping is reminiscent of the fun we had with friends on the playground.[3] V   4 V

Using Arms and Hands

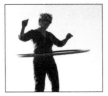
When I first learned to hoop, like most people, I struck the pose affectionately referred to as the "T. rex," in which we position our arms and hands like an upright dinosaur or sentinel groundhog. Caroleeena has studied flamenco, Indian classical, Bollywood, hula, modern, and belly dance. The first thing she considers in hoopdance is carriage, the way we distribute our weight throughout the muscular-skeletal system for movement. If you consciously break the

T. rex pose by shifting your awareness from the hoop to your arms and hands, you will move more freely while hoopdancing.

Learning to move your hands and arms gracefully is a matter of practicing new patterns. Once you are comfortable with a pattern, it becomes second nature, and you can incorporate it into any routine at any time. Caroleeena's online tutorial for an across-the-chest hoop roll is a good example of practicing a hand pattern.[5] V

You can use your hands to rotate the hoop vertically in front of you, horizontally around the body, or above the head like a lasso. Miss Rosie, creator of Movement Play in California, introduced me to the "lobster claw" at a class she offered in Berkeley. The idea is to guide momentum with gentle hand control, keeping the thumb on one side of the hoop and fingers on the other, in a grasp-and-push motion.

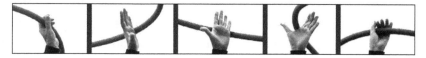

Another way to guide the hoop with your hand, or some other part of your body, is to "stall" it. Vivian Hancock (Spiral), who brought hooping to Carrboro, North Carolina, says, "When you perform a hoop stall during lifts and other plane transfers, you sync up your speed with the hoop's to keep open a 'window of opportunity,' or space in the center of the hoop. This adds both ease and grace." Ease, because synchronizing velocity slows down the apparent time needed to get from one impulse to the next, and grace, because the extra time allows you to relax into the move. The hoop doesn't stop turning in a stall, rather your hand or whole body matches its rate of speed so 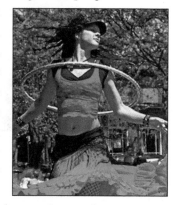 that the hoop appears to be nearly stationary. Stall the hoop on your chest by turning your body at the same speed and in the same direction as the hoop, with shoulders down and arms stretching back.

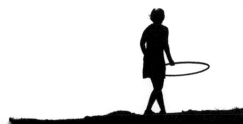

Explore the space in and around your hoop with your hands and arms before you try fancy tricks and twirls. Try using either hand to stall the hoop while it is traveling around your waist. Take it from one hip to the other by holding it away from your body for a second, with the palm or back of your hand matching its speed and direction. Diana Lopez (BodyHoops) plays with the full range of where her hands can be at any given moment. She dips them in and out, and reaches beyond the hoop on both sides, in front, and in back in a ten-minute playful workout.[6] V

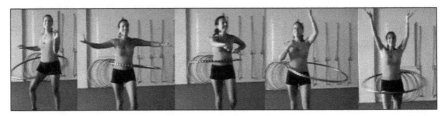

As you practice, you will discover many ways to move with the hoop, some of them all your own. Remember to stay hydrated, to be mindful of posture at all times, and to bring energy up from your feet and down from your shoulders into the core. If you challenge yourself, the hoop will fall, which will make you laugh, and laughter is a medicinal property of your hoop. Make one today and get started. (More about hoops in chapter 9.)

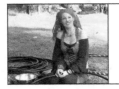
Eco Faeries show you how to make a recycled hoop from irrigation tubing.[7] V

Making a Hoop

To make adult-size hoops you can use one-inch, three-quarter-inch, or half-inch, 160- or 100-psi irrigation tubing. I buy mine at a local landscape irrigation supply store. To find material in your area, try building supply outlets, search the Internet for "irrigation tubing [your city and state]," or check the make-your-own section at PsiHoops.com.

Psi, pounds per square inch, refers to the amount of water pressure the tubing can withstand. Higher psi tubing is heavier.

Barbed-plastic internal connectors are sold in many hardware and garden irrigation supply stores; a ratcheting PVC cutter is useful for cutting the tubing to the lengths you need, but you can also use a saw. To estimate the appropriate length of tubing for the hoop size you want to end up with, multiply the desired diameter (for instance, the distance from the floor to your breastbone) by 3.14 (mathematical *pi*) and cut a length of tubing to that size. For a hoop that stands vertical at approximately 42 inches, the length of tubing needed is 132 inches, or 11 feet.

Use a hair dryer, or a pan of boiled water, to heat and soften one end of the tubing. Insert it over one half of the connector. Then soften the other end of the tubing and push it over the other half of the connector. Voilà, you've made a hoop that is ready to decorate with tape.

A single line of gaffer tape or a bit of roughing up with sand paper along the inner side of the hoop is all you need to add traction; the rest is personal style. One-inch- and half-inch-wide tapes work best. Smooth and slick ones go down first, with textured types added on top for traction. Websites like Identi-Tape.com have holographic, glow-in-the-dark, glitter, and gaffer tape in every color, style, and size imaginable. (See the Resources section at the back of the book.)

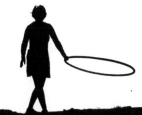

Spike and gaffer tapes have a tacky surface, making the hoop easier to use because it grips. Theater, photo, or cinema supply stores carry these tapes in a range of colors and patterns.

Electrical tape is the cheapest, smoothest, and easiest to apply. It comes in bright colors at hardware and drug stores.

Metallic tapes come in many colors with a slippery surface. Genuine copper tape can be found in the garden-pest department of hardware stores and nurseries.

Cork bicycle-handlebar tape, available at cycle shops and on the Internet, creates a durable, cushioned, but expensive alternative.

Warm-up Exercises

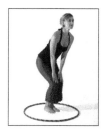 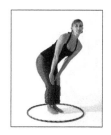 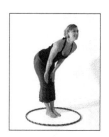 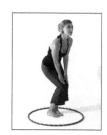

1. Ankles and Knees: Using your hoop as a guide on the floor, stand at its center and place your feet close together. Keep the outer sides of your feet parallel, which may feel a bit pigeon-toed. Place your hands on slightly bent knees. Use the muscles along the inner side of your legs to draw energy up from the arch of your foot to your solar plexus, creating an axis around which to move. Flex your ankles and feel your weight shift around all the edges of your feet as you make slow circles. Make seven circles in one direction and then seven in the opposite.

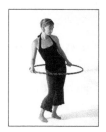 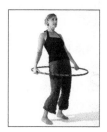 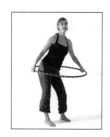 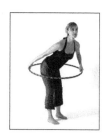

2. Hips: Pick up your hoop, keeping knees slightly bent. Place feet hip-width apart, so that your thigh and shinbones make a straight line from hip to ankle. Begin to trace the inner circle of the hoop with your hips. Keep your alignment as stationary as possible while making wide circles. Swivel your hips and rib cage around the imaginary axis that runs from the center of your head, through the center of the hoop, and into the floor between the arches of your feet. Keep the triangle of each foot firmly

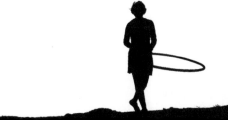

planted, drawing energy up through the arches along the inside of each leg. Energize your ankles and knees, but move from your core. Repeat seven rotations in each direction, noting any points of resistance that need gentle coaxing. As in learning to hoopdance, there is no need to hurry your warm-up.

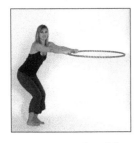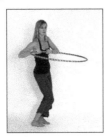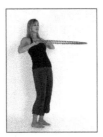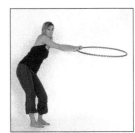

3. Shoulders and Arms: With feet hip-width apart and knees flexed, use a lightweight hoop to stretch out in front of you, moving it opposite to your hips, as if you are stirring a pot with the center point of your hoop. The pelvis goes back and the rib cage comes forward as the hoop stretches out in front. Hips go left, ribs right, as you reach to the right. Pelvis pushes forward as you pull the hoop in close to your chest, rounding your back. Hips go right, ribs left, as you reach to the left. Pelvis pushes back again as you stretch arms and chest in front again. Complete seven of these expansive circles in each direction.

To do this with a partner, use a larger hoop between you. As you pull the hoop in toward your chest, your partner will push outward. When you go left, your partner goes right, and so forth, seven times in each direction.

Basic Waist Hooping

Extending the hoop's momentum to keep it spinning around the core involves timing and proper muscle use, but oddly enough it is not a circular motion or twist. The basic thrust comes from your core, between the collarbone and thighs. Hooping Harmony's Laura Marie says, "You need to have both feet pointing forward and make sure your hips aren't cocked at an odd angle. Pelvis is squared off forward. Don't go rigid in your knees, because you need a little bit of softness there."

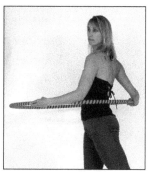

- To begin, place one foot slightly forward of the other.
- Place the hoop at the small of the back, and wind up in a twist to one side.
- Use your forearms to level the hoop, and then give it a good strong push with both hands to get it moving.
- Immediately begin to push from your core as the hoop makes contact with the body front and back, drawing energy up through your feet and legs.

If you have never hooped before, or someone you are teaching can't seem to do it immediately, try getting a feel for the timing of the hoop's revolution before trying to keep it going. To do this, begin as above by placing the hoop at the small of the back, twisting to one side, and giving a strong push, *but* don't try to make contact. Just stand still and let the hoop rotate. Feel the way it moves. Keep doing this until the hoop stays level and moves around on its own momentum for a few revolutions. Then try again to keep it going.

Once you can hoop with one foot a little ahead of the other, switch to the other foot forward, pumping front to back. Then try it with feet evenly set beneath the hips and pulse side to side. Alternate these stances in every practice, and spin the hoop in both directions.

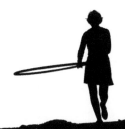

Stretching

After hooping, stretch to prevent muscle stiffness and discomfort.

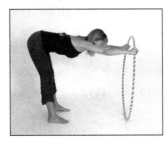 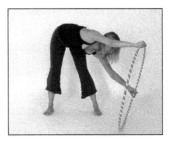

- Hold the hoop vertically in front of you without putting much pressure on it. Bend forward from the hips with a flat back, and lengthen the back of the legs to release tension. Slowly roll the hoop to each side, lengthening the sides of the body and relaxing the head.

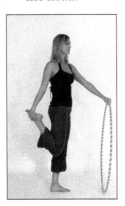 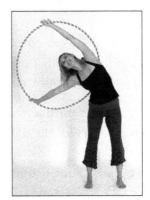 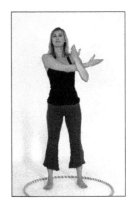

- Using the hoop for balance, grasp each foot in turn from behind. Pointing the knee toward the floor will lengthen the thigh.
- Hold the hoop behind your upper body and stretch the sides of your body as you bend to each side, keeping the chest open.
- Stretch your shoulders by bringing each arm in front of your chest and adding a little pressure until you feel a stretch over your back shoulder blade.
- Then shake out your head, neck, and limbs.

Chapter Two Links

www.HoopDanceBook.com/chapter2

1. *Ashrita Furman Interview.* Nov. 28, 2009.
2. *Caroleeena on Hoop Consciousness.* Jun. 29, 2009.
3. *FlowShow2: Remembering Recess.* Apr. 30, 2010.
4. *The Hoopers' Playground.* Mar. 1, 2012.
5. *Hand Flip for Across the Chest Hoop Roll.* Nov. 6, 2009.
6. *Hula Hoop with BodyHoops 10 minute workout.* Sep. 29, 2009.
7. *How to Make a Hula Hoop.* Jun. 5, 2011.

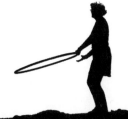

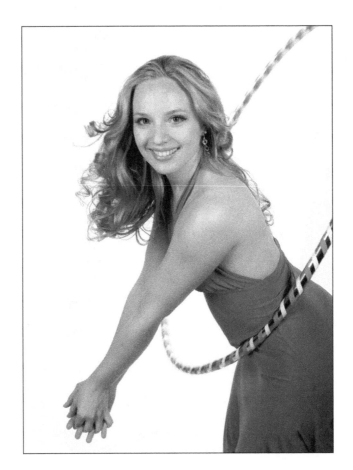

Laura Marie angle hooping

THREE

Beyond the Basics

Ain't nothin' good unless you play with it.
—George Clinton, singer/songwriter

Inspired by Hooping Harmony in Massachusetts, I wanted to meet everyone who was making hoopdance a life choice. I started by contacting
Christabel Zamor, because she trained most of the teachers I took classes
with in Berkeley. Christabel introduced me to Rich Porter and Khan
Wong. Rich introduced me to Brecken Rivara and Beth Lavinder. Thus
began my journey, where the influence of these and many other marvel-
ous hoopers took me to the next level of my own practice. Their stories
and tips give us a further glimpse into the hoopdance movement's form
and philosophy.

Lifting Off and Moving Around

Once we master the basic biomechanics involved in handling a hoop,
style emerges in the way we walk and turn, make lines with our bodies, and trace patterns with our hoops. Taking classes with a variety of
hoopdancers who were trained in the same program, I noticed that each
teacher had his or her own unique way of thinking about movement and
executing tricks. With several teachers I learned several versions of "lasso,"
lifting the hoop from the waist to revolve it above my head. It can be done
with one or both arms. The one-arm method requires a change in the lifting hand that is useful to master on your way to more advanced dancing.

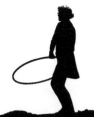

Here's how it goes:

- If you are hooping to the right (clockwise), use the left hand to lift. For hooping to the left (counterclockwise), use your right. Whichever you start with is your first hand.

- Place your first hand against the back of your waist, palm facing out.

- When you feel the hoop rolling over your first hand, lift it around to the front and into the air with a loose touch, letting your elbow guide the hoop straight up in front of your face as you turn with small, stable steps in the hoop's direction.

- Your palm remains open to change, and your thumb ends up on the other side of the hoop.[1] V

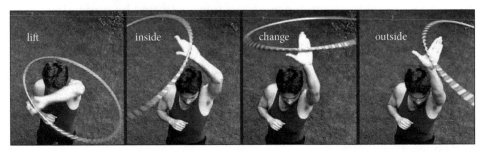

To accomplish this move I had to guide and interact with the hoop more freely, relinquishing my lobster-claw, grip-and-push control. Practicing without the hoop helped. Imagine a cup of tea sitting in the palm of your first hand as you place it against your back. Now bring that imaginary teacup straight up and around past your face, without spilling, to hold it above your head as you turn in the same direction as your hoop. Notice that the hand must change orientation in order to keep the cup upright.

Once you learn to guide the hoop from your waist to above your head, you can bring it back down. The lifting hand keeps the hoop moving while the other sneaks into the circle and glides the hoop down to the waist, giving it a sturdy push toward the back when it gets there. Lifting the hoop with the first hand and guiding it down with the second can be practiced independently. Then you can put them together to create a seamless vortex of spirals as you turn in the direction of the hoop while repeatedly guiding it up from the waist to above the head and back down again.

Become the Line

Each gesture or transition we make while hoopdancing creates a visual line. There is a big difference between lifting the hoop from the waist to above the head with your arm fully extended, and leaving a bend at the elbow with the hoop just clearing the top of the head. The extra extension creates a beautiful line as well as a successful lift. The dancer's lines follow the way his or her body posture and limbs extend into space. They

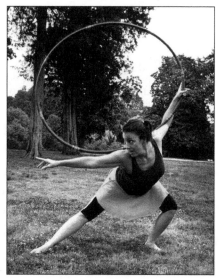

describe the way we use the space around us while hoopdancing. Instructor Caroleeena says, "We create the illusion of an even longer line by focusing our gaze slightly *beyond* fully extended fingertips and toes. That makes us look and feel taller, thinner, and more striking."

In contrast, if you want a line that appears to stop short, use a flexed hand, foot, arm, leg, or torso. When Caroleeena performs an eagle roll, with the hoop rolling over her back from one extended hand to the other, several lines appear. The longest one is made from her backward extending arm to the forward extending leg. The next longest follows both arms, and the line from head through chest to leg is stopped short by a bent knee. The result is a strikingly elegant pose with counterpoint.

Staying aware of body lines is a common quandary for hoopdancers. For instance, when one hand is lifting the hoop off the body, the secondary arm tends to take the fallback T. rex position, with a bent elbow causing a bump in the overall line from hoop to toes. To smooth the line, we can include the secondary arm in the movement. Drop the hand to rest gently against a leg, tuck it behind the back, or let it trace the energy of the hoop's path.

In yoga we learn to drop the body into the floor, pressing our feet down, while simultaneously lifting up to press the top of the head upward. As you

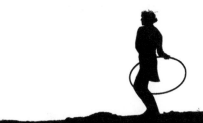

learn to hoopdance, think about extending your body in every direction, lengthening your neck, and completing lines with your chin and the crown of your head. Lifting the rib cage—front, back, and sides—not only helps you create beautiful lines but it also relieves pressure on bones and joints, and frees your core for its full range of motion. This requires gluteal and lower abdominal muscles to be engaged, shoulders and knees relaxed. Experiment in front of a mirror or videotape yourself to see how many variations of lines you can create with arms and legs in different transitions while moving. Notice how subtle posture changes can lengthen or shorten your appearance in space.

The First Step

Hula hooping and many of its tricks can be accomplished standing in one spot, but moving is essential to prevent repetitive strain. Traveling steps allow us to move about and turn, which is essential for smooth transitions with striking lines, but taking your first steps may be awkward, especially if you are new to isolating your core. Before you start walking, bounce without the hoop from one foot to the other, feeling your weight shift evenly from your center to each side. Then, when you are in the hoop, you can let your body and the hoop's momentum tell you when to use a shift of weight or a bounce with a traveling step.

Individual steps can be practiced for quite some time before putting them together in a stride. While waist hooping, three things will help you walk and turn: (1) use abdominal muscles more precisely to free your motion, (2) push more firmly into the hoop just prior to stepping, and (3) remember that the energy activating your hoop comes from the ground up, always lifting.

To take your first step:

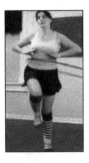

- Start to waist hoop with one foot in front of the other. Imagine your naval moving toward the spine. Breathe into the motion.
- Feel the propulsive rhythm. Engage your midsection. And shift your weight to the front foot while stepping the other forward.
- Put down the stepping foot firmly, regain your rhythm, and redistribute your weight.
- Shift into the next step with the other foot.[2] Ⅴ

After taking steps, learn to walk, and then practice stepping high while hooping, and even jumping, to develop balance. Put as much effort as possible into creating shifts in direction and height early on; dip down to cross one foot in front of and then behind the other, stand tall, and walk backwards and sideways to create dynamic movement.

Learn to Turn

Turning makes everything smoother in hoopdance, but it may cause some people to become dizzy, so start slowly. The dancers' technique of "spotting," which uses gaze to stabilize the horizon, can help. I learned it this way: focus on a stationary object over one shoulder, and pivot halfway around to focus on the same object over the other shoulder. If you take a step with each pivot, you can half-turn continuously to travel a length of ground.

Turning in the same direction as your hoop slows your movement down, giving you more time to get into and out of position. Turning in the direction opposite to your hoop's movement speeds it up, which is useful for variation. The two types of steps I use most are small stable ones for sustained spinning (turning continuously without pause), or a pivot on the ball of one foot while pushing with the other for a full turn in one swift movement.

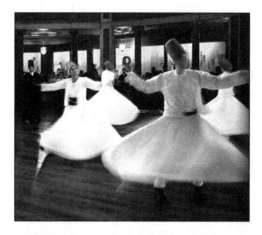

Whirling dervishes, spinning dancers
of Sufism, stay grounded while turning
by using a series of stable steps.

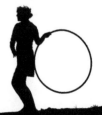

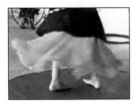

Julia Hartsell (Jewels), creator of the annual Hoop Convergence event in North Carolina, starts with feet parallel. She steps one foot out to form a wide V, with heels staying close together, and then steps with the other foot to bring the toes close, with heels apart.[3] [V]

You can also turn gracefully with the hoop held off-body. Betty Lucas specializes in teaching Hoop Chi, combining ballroom dance steps with Tai Chi moves to create sequences like her "tango turn."[4] [V]

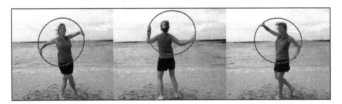

Build on Trust

A chance meeting and shared interest in the creative potential of hoopdance are often all that one hooper needs to believe in another. Trust sometimes falters, and betrayals can happen, but giving each other (and ourselves) the benefit of the doubt comes naturally with the hoop. When I planned my research trip around the eastern third of the United States, hoopers put me up all along the way. When I found someone interesting on the Internet, I got in touch by e-mail, was always invited to visit, and was usually offered a place to stay. Something similar happened when Christabel Zamor (HoopGirl) met Rayna McInturf (Hoopnotica) and was invited to stay with her in Los Angeles.

Christabel teaches walking and turning while hooping and balancing an empty plastic cup or water-filled balloon on her head. (Try it to see what

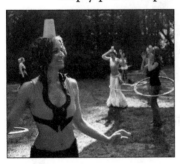

adding a prop does for your posture.) Author of the workout manual *Hooping: A Revolutionary Fitness Program,* Christabel says, "Hooping can catapult your sex life to the next level. You build incredible core strength, tone and slim the belly and buttocks, develop better hand-eye coordination, and unwind the spine. What does all this mean? Your confidence soars." But she was not always so self-assured.

Christabel had been a pudgy, shy, cigarette smoking, anthropology student without much self-esteem when she saw Rayna hoopdancing at the Beltane/May Day music festival in Ojai, California. Rayna took Christabel under her wing and introduced her to Anah Reichenbach (Hoopalicious) in Los Angeles. The mutual trust of these three women went a long way to further the development of hoopdance.

When Christabel took her first hoopdance work-shop, she couldn't keep the hoop up. "I tried and tried. While everyone else in the class was beautiful and spec-tacular, moving like fairies or otherworldly graceful beings, I was clumsy and frustrated." Nonetheless she bought a hoop and started practicing on the beach.[5] V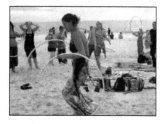

People wanted to know what she was doing; she got them hooping. They wanted hoops; she made hoops. They wanted classes; she started teaching. Then opportunities to perform presented themselves, and she blossomed. She founded the performance troupe HoopGirl AllStars and the first teacher training program for hoopdance to be approved by the Aerobics and Fitness Association of America.

After receiving two master's degrees, one in cultural anthropology and the other in mythological studies, Christabel trained in somatic education, became a licensed white-belt nia instructor, as well as a zumba fitness instructor (two hybrid dance-exercise modalities), and a "laughter" yoga teacher (using self-triggered laughing for deep diaphragm breathing). She founded HoopGirl as a company in 2001 and certified more than six hun-dred instructors in sixteen countries.

Off-Body Isolations

Hoop "isolation" refers to manipulation around a point in space rather than a part of your body. The hoop appears to remain stationary. Imagine the steering wheel turning in your car. Your hands and arms move the wheel while it stays in place, turning around a central point.

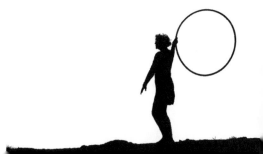

Jocelyn Gordon calls the center point of an isolation the *drishti* point, in reference to the yogic concept of eye focus. Creator of HoopYogini, she

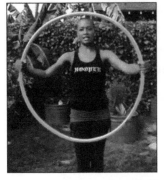

shares her integrative perspective on hooping through online classes and international retreats. Hooping represents everything she loves: it is a massage for her organs and lymphatic system, a mindfulness practice like yoga, and her free-form style of dance. Originally from Bermuda, she came to California by way of Washington, D.C., where she founded Hoop Dance DC and was an active member of the DC Hoop Collective. In California she became a Hoopnotica master trainer and is a former director of the Hoopnotica teacher-training program.

Exploring "outside" isolations, Jocelyn shows us how to grip the hoop with one hand, moving it from top to bottom and back again, while the other hand traces the action on the hoop's opposite side. "Outside-hoop isolations discover the curve of the hoop and then extend that curve out into different directions." She identifies the "mother hand" (to move the hoop) and the "tracing hand" (to follow the curve on the other side).[6] V

To learn the more difficult one-handed, inside-hoop isolation that Jocelyn demonstrates at the beginning of her video, two things are helpful:

1. Try practicing the pattern of the movement while a friend holds a hoop stationary on the vertical plane in front of you. Move your whole arm and shoulder to trace an inside grip around the circle of the hoop. Notice that your hand must flip at the top in order to trace, and eventually guide, the hoop back down the other side.

2. When you actually move the hoop in a stationary full circle, keep the edges of the hoop in all four quadrants of your peripheral vision as you softly focus on the *drishti* point. Frame something with the hoop, and try to keep it centered. Practice in front of a mirror to see how your arm and shoulder work to create the illusion in space. As you master isolations, dancing as you move the hoop enhances the visual effect.

It's not surprising that men, with their greater upper body strength, would add new territory to the land of hoopdance with off-body forms, nor that women would be quick to follow. These moves are fun to watch and to perform. They are a great way to limber, stretch, and strengthen shoulders, arms, and wrists.

Isopop

Intrigued by the videos Rich Porter posted on his Isopop website, I e-mailed him with an introduction from Christabel. He suggested we meet for lunch near his office in San Francisco. This was my first in-person interview, and I was excited by the prospect of meeting one of my heroes. I allowed plenty of extra travel time, arrived early, and sat in the sun outside the restaurant to wait. Would I recognize him? I thought Rich might look quite different on the city streets from his performance on the Internet, but there was no mistaking the figure waiting for the light to change while talking on his mobile phone. Even from a distance the short bleached hair, muscular yet 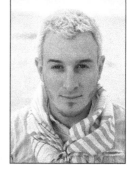 sinuous body language, and the modest way he walked let me know it was Rich. We took our lunch to a table in the park, and I tested my new digital recorder. I wanted to know everything. He started by telling me that an "isopop" is hoop isolation with a visual "pop."

When you are tracing a circle with a hoop as an inside isolation, if you stop your arm rotation and release the hoop, it will continue to move around your hand on its own momentum. Resume the isolation by grasping it again when it regains the same position in which you let it go. The effect is dramatic, as if the hoop pops out of the isolation and back in again.

Rich was instrumental in advancing the technique of hoop isolations, but he didn't join the movement on impulse. In 2006 he was working as an architectural designer in San Luis Obispo, one of California's hooping hot spots, when his wife, Lauren (Onyx), saw hoopdancing at raves in Los Angeles. She wanted to do it, so Rich helped her make a hoop from instructions on the Internet. "I just

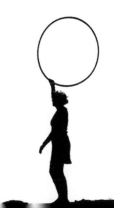

watched at first," he says, "but eventually it became something we did together." They met other hoopers and spinners in the park, where Rich found men with whom to practice and develop his hooping style. Learning led to teaching and performance.[7] [V]

Spinning

Object manipulation with a variety of props, such as the hoop, is referred to as "spinning." Swinging a pair of balls on cords around the body to create visual patterns is called "spinning *poi*," a Maori practice from New Zealand. While hoopdancing is kinesthetic, learned by reactions within the body, spinning engages logic and has specific language for developing technique. Rich used an architectural approach to think out patterns for the hoop in the way that spinners do for *poi*. "If you understand spinning terminology and I say 'split time, same direction, anti-spin flowers' you know exactly the moves I am talking about and what they look like."

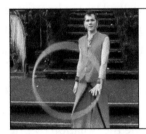

Rainbow Michaels explains that moving the hoop opposite to the direction of the hooper's shoulder is called "anti-spin flowers."[8] [V]

In Rich's search for language that could bring the same transparency to hooping that he found in the spinning community, he attended a HoopPath workshop taught by the program's founder, Jonathan Baxter. During the first class Rich was mystified by the stories of an ancient culture that Baxter used to explain the movement he demonstrated. How could Rich have missed learning about the Maidan (pronounced "myDAN") in his college coursework? He found no information in reference books or online because Baxter had invented the Maidan himself. When Rich began to develop the Hoop Technique training program, terminology from Baxter's way of teaching helped him name the steps in his own process for off-body hooping.

The genealogy of hoopdance is revealed in the language we use to speak about movement and the ways in which we dance. Rich says, "Where you learn leaves an indelible mark. You can see regional differences among early hoopdancers." The community of friends he started hooping with included spinners, and more men than women. That influenced his style. Every hooper has a who-made-you story, but eventually each person's hooping style becomes unique, the way fingerprints differentiate us from each other.

Boulder, Colorado's Nick Guzzardo was exposed to a mixture of influences at international events when he started hooping. His dancing exhibits a unique amalgamation of moves. Hints of Rich Porter and Beth Lavinder's off-body moves, Baxter's breaking, Karis' flare, and Anah Reichenbach's dancing merge with his own exploration of the hoop.[9] V

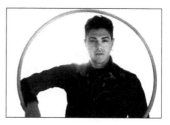

Alternating Currents

Beth Lavinder started hooping in the innovative atmosphere of Carrboro, North Carolina. In 2003 she saw Spiral on the lawn at the Weaver Street Market co-op. "I couldn't take my eyes off her. It felt voyeuristic, and I was captivated by something very sensuous and beautiful." Beth was delighted that she could keep a hoop spinning when she tried it herself, because she had never before thought of herself as graceful. Eventually she joined a HoopPath class, and her own style began to emerge.

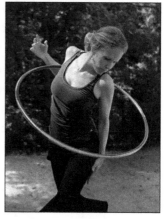

Watching Spiral gave Beth a glimpse of what was possible; Baxter's HoopPath philosophy gave her the meaning she needed in order to work through challenges and learn to hoopdance. "In what we call a 'first tree break' I reach across my midline to catch the hoop on the far end of my reach and bring it back over. This is uncomfortable, but I do it because the more I practice what is awkward, the more I develop ease and grace." In HoopPath terminology everything Beth learned about hooping in her "first current" (easier direction) was rearticulated in her less natural "second current."

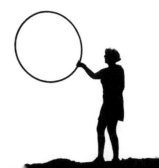

It reminded Beth of learning Japanese when she was twenty-seven years old. After studying and practicing architecture in the United States, she lived in northern Japan and married a Japanese man. She had no choice but to be immersed in a second language. "Each word had to go through translation from my natural first language to the one in which I was less at ease."

Mastering your second current gives you the power to reverse the hoop's direction on any plane, on any part of the body, or while swinging it around off-body and overhead. Reversals add both challenge and excitement, but notice that an odd number of reversals will bring you continually back to your comfort zone. The key is to balance movement in your more natural first current with the same move in your more difficult second. To master reverses, practice mirroring every movement with its opposite for a song or two each time you practice. You may have to devote a whole day or even an entire week to hooping in your awkward direction before becoming bilingual in your movement. If you start hooping in both directions from the beginning, the translation from one direction to another will be in your brain, bones, and viscera.

As a warm-up drill, I like to spin the hoop around my waist in one direction for four or five revolutions, stop the hoop by grasping it on two sides when it is against my back, and, keeping it level, reverse its direction for another four or five revolutions. Imagine doing that continuously as fast as you can while dancing for three or four songs at a time. You will get comfortable with the idea of reversals in no time. Then you can add flourish, do it one-handed, or use the inside of your forearm to bounce the hoop into the opposite direction no matter where it is.

In Japan Beth had a Shinto wedding and became fluent in Japanese, but after five years she still felt like an outsider. She fit into the culture well in some ways and would never fit in others. When she came back to North Carolina, hooping helped her readjust as she practiced architecture, deepened her marriage, and relished being a mother. Then teaching presented itself as the next challenge. It changed her role from a hoopdancer participating in a learning process within a circle of friends to a more public figure of authority. At Hoopcamp she taught her peers. "It was a surreal experience to be with the people I adore, in the sea of their energy, and presume to teach them what I knew."

Whether as a student or teacher, Beth brings an understanding of both strength and gentleness to hoopdance. She doesn't try to hoop like anybody else, not as beautifully as Spiral, nor as athletically as Baxter. Much like jazz musicians playing together, hoopdancers, rather than mimic each other, inspire one another through hooping conversations in which different points of view and perspectives are shared.

When Beth dances, her body rises up to meet the hoop and dips down to follow it in micro-movements. She approaches each hoop revolution as a wave that becomes an expression that builds on the next. She can't imagine life without hoopdance. "When I move the hoop up into a crest, down into the trough, and then back up that might be a phrase. If I gather phrases, they become sentences, and sentences become paragraphs. If I do this long enough, I'm going to have a really sweet chapter and I might even have a novel in the end. When I'm eighty, I hope I'm still moving with the hoop in whatever way is possible." [10] [V]

Breaking Planes

Just as reversals bring the hoop from one direction to another, hooping transitions can bring the hoop from one plane to another. Brecken Rivara came to the hoopdance scene with unconventional transitions between horizontal, vertical, and diagonal planes. She wasn't focused on performance, but she moved with a physical genius that attracted the hooping community's notice. [11] [V]

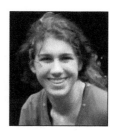

Rich and Christabel brought Brecken from the East Coast to San Francisco to teach two classes at the Margaret Jenkins Dance Lab. I met her at the first class. She arrived breathless and harried in a T-shirt and sweats, and we sat on the floor talking in the hallway as her students entered with their sparkling hoops. In class she was unassuming. Her loose clothing covered smooth muscles that revealed themselves as she stretched and lengthened her limbs.

Brecken illustrated, to hoopers more accomplished than I, an approach to creating transitions through personal imagery. Many teachers stress

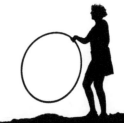

directing attention inward to an awareness of the body. She suggested that we go a step further to project the body's "feeling impulses," the urges that drive the way we move, outward to imagined surroundings. "Create an atmosphere in which to be compelled," she directed. "Imagine a terrain of hills, water, clouds—anything to which you can tangibly react. Then be dropped and pulled by your imagination as a servant of the music."

Brecken's body lines extend into space like emotional highways. When her movements are kept small and in place, they convey timidity; then stretching into larger lines, she conveys a feeling of boldness. In her second class, "Poise & Finesse," I learned to channel my breath into the lines I created with my body and to control my hoop with elongation, lightness, and torque—alternately swinging it away from me and then quickly pulling it back into isolation.

Inspired by modern dance, Brecken encouraged us to pair explosive movements with intimate ones and to learn from our own experience. Paradoxically, she doesn't feel that poise and finesse can actually be taught. "Eventually through trial and error," she says, "I figure out one little piece of a movement to work from; then I keep reworking it until it becomes a part of my hooping style. The hoop is the real teacher." Her *Eye of the Storm* video is overlaid with stream-of-consciousness narration to reveal her process of impulse, trial, error, and persistence.[12] [V]

Brecken came to hooping with an artist's desire to communicate. In college she studied painting and acting. "I was obsessed with realistic painting, but at some point I got discouraged that I wasn't expressing myself, so I tried acting. I took a lead role in a play and worked very hard at conveying various emotions, becoming different characters, but that was equally dismal." She left school in Baltimore and went home to New Jersey to simply do nothing for a while. Then a friend came to visit and gave her a big hoop.

Brecken got pretty good at hooping even though she only played with it occasionally. One day, closing her eyes, she experienced what she calls "the silliness of it." She began following the hoop with her feelings rather than trying to accomplish something. The freedom of not having to show anyone what she was doing released her creativity and allowed something real to happen. "I gave up trying to show what I could do. I expected nothing. Working for the art form alone rather than for validation of myself, discoveries with the hoop became endless."

Activities that allow us to experience what we already know in a new or unusual way, just to satisfy curiosity with our minds at rest, lead to creative learning and bring about elated feelings. Brecken understands the creative process (submitting, asserting, and following), which supersedes the specific form of any artistic activity. Merging her intentions with the hoop's momentum, her body lines are built out of necessity, based on what she feels most urgently moved to do. "The intention to articulate energy with an arm eventually elongates the arm because the intention requires it. Then because it is practiced so often, it becomes a characteristic of your body. As you work to translate something bigger than yourself, energy is transmuted into a form that others can experience."

Hooping for its own sake, discovering your true self—how you feel, listen, and find beauty—parallels other art disciplines.

Brecken attributes innovation to personal exploration rather than formal training, and she advises new hoopdancers not to take classes for a couple of years. "What you invest yourself in dictates your style, so the novice has a certain advantage, a clean slate. On your own, the move you intend to make is up to you. You simply have to find your own way to do it."

Simple Plane Transfers and Weaves

An early Hoopalicious tutorial introduces the idea of transferring the hoop from the horizontal plane to the diagonal around the waist. To do the "barrel roll," you must bend slightly forward with flexed knees and bounce to keep the hoop in motion, and then turn in the direction of the hoop, bending sideways and backward to stay with the angle of the hoop, pumping to keep it on the diagonal plane all the while.[13] V

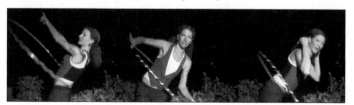

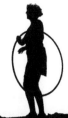

Using the diagonal plane off-body, Emma Kerr's Hooping Mad tutorial gets you started with a figure eight and a jump. When you jump into the hoop from an off-body maneuver, you can either toss it onto your core or bring it up over your head for another off-body move. As you articulate a fairly flat figure eight with your arm and hand, the hoop draws it three-dimensionally in space.

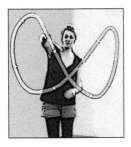

Begin with the hoop vertical at your side, holding the top loosely, palm up. Then twist it up and over diagonally in front of you, to swing down by your other side, palm now on the top of the hoop. Lift it with another twist of the wrist to swing back over to its original position. You can jump through the hoop either sideways as it comes toward center, or straight on by swinging it toward your feet in front.[14] V

Beats and Weaves

A figure eight has two beats, one for each side of the swing. A weave is a figure eight done with two hoops crossing each other, one in each hand. A three-beat weave lets the hoop revolve around the hand at one side for the third beat. When Sharna Rose posted a tutorial of her five-beat weave, it caused a sensation on YouTube.

Sharna had fostered hoopdancing in England by starting the U.K. Hoop Dance Tribe on the Internet and videotaping her experiments. She invites others to ask, "What if we do this?" or say, "I reckon you could do that." Gail O'Brien, founder of the Manchester Hoop Congress, says, "Sharna has been hooping the longest in our community, and she has no agenda or drive to block the openness of the hoopdance culture she started."

Sharna says, "It's like a snowball rolling down a long mountain slope. Our community expands and grows." She is a hoop maker, performer, and certified hoopdance instructor, but before taking classes with U.S. hoopers Diana Lopez (BodyHoops) and Christabel Zamor (HoopGirl), she developed her own unique style in southeast England, where she lives with her husband and children. "Stay true to who you are because that is your gift to the world," she advises. "Learn at your own speed, and allow your whole body to move with each rotation of the hoop. Be soft, gentle, yielding, and bouncy." She perfects the things that feel wrong, or the opposite of what she is trying to do, into a new routine, quoting Hoopalicious to say, "The mistakes of today are tomorrow's moves."

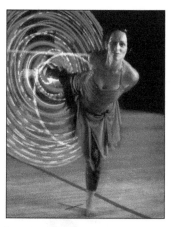

Sharna describes herself as "a mildly obsessive-compulsive Libra," so hooping in both directions was natural for her from the start, and she credits her best work to a craving for balance. After she threw herself into yoga, the gym, and swimming, only to become bored with each, a year of ecstatic dancing brought out her true identity. "Dancing like a crazy thing makes me feel connected to the chaotic balance of the universe, like the flower child of hippie parents that I am."

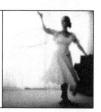

Sharna dances to
"We Are All Connected."[15] V

To do her five-beat weave, Sharna added a jump-through and a toss to a three-beat weave as the fourth and fifth beats. Her version is a hybrid of the five-beat weave done with *poi*, which was considered impossible to do with hoops until Steve Bags posted his tutorial of the intricate trick. Bags color-codes his hoops and shirtsleeves to help us keep track of them, and gives time code in his video so that his technique can be reviewed in individual steps.[16] V

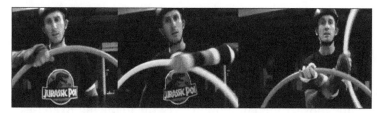

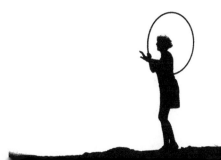

Playing in Place

On a less technical note, Sandra Summerville (SaFire) gives bonus points for making airplane noises while hooping. She founded HoopCity.ca, an

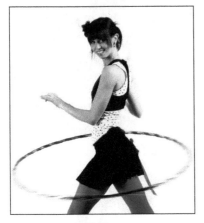

online space for hoopers, in Alberta, Canada. She considers trying to avoid awkwardness to be a road filled with ruts. Her remedy? "Be as ridiculous as you can. Wonderful things can happen when we take advantage of opportunities to be silly." At an international children's festival, SaFire was stepping out of her hoop when she noticed that her shoelace was untied. She decided to see if she could tie it while hooping on one leg. The kids went wild. One-legged hooping looks cool, and seeing SaFire tie a shoe while doing it was even better. "Mix it up," she advises, "hoop who you are, and multitask."

Reading a book helped SaFire learn to knee hoop because she was diverted from thinking about controlling the hoop. Try eating an ice cream cone or enjoying a hot drink while hooping. My husband, Tom, and I take a break in the hoop most days. We work from our home, so at coffee time we put the iPod player in the doorway, take our cups into the street, where spillage has minor consequences on the pavement, and hoop for three songs. Hooping with a cup of hot liquid may seem like a silly challenge, but it changes the energy whether you are waist hooping or trying not to spill as you lasso, single weave, and jump.

You can change speed and size to vary any routine, slow or fast, big or small. For instance, in passing a hoop around the body, SaFire says, "We can keep it tight like little lemons, or we can stretch it out and become as big as lions. Same move, different motion." Try the following Exercises à la SaFire both slowly and quickly, and taking up a little or a lot of space.

To emulate a Flash Mob, just flood a public place with hoopdancers for three minutes (as Emma did in Brighton) and then disperse at once.[17] [V]

Exercises à la SaFire

Obstacle hooping. SaFire believes in grounding all of our hoop play in "dynamic space," seeing the environment as alive with possibility and changing constantly as we move through it. Playing with obstacles gives us a creative challenge. The idea is to move as fluidly as possible. You, the hoop, and the obstacle are at play. In his movies, martial arts star Jackie Chan uses whatever is available to outwit his opponents. Choreographing a fight in a restaurant, he may hurl chairs and cups. In a train station he will leap over tracks and hang from trestles. Urban gymnasts call this *le parkour* or "park core." They jump up walls, flip off buildings, and slither under railings. You can use the furniture in your house, trees and rocks in nature, or poles, curbing, and stairs in town. Pass your hoop around things; go under and over them.

Patty cake. Agree on a pattern of hand touching with a friend who may or may not be hooping. Play the pattern while you hoop. If you've had a late night, this one might boggle the mind a bit, but multitasking to isolate the mind and body can prepare you to take on more complex moves with the hoop.

Hoop hopscotch. Practice to jump and land on your feet while hooping. Lay several hoops out in a meandering path with a little space between each consecutive hoop. The aim of the game is to jump from the center of one hoop to another while core hooping. Doing this with a group adds the challenge of paying attention to the pace of your fellow hoopers.

Limitations. Hoopers often talk about running out of new things to do to fend off boredom. In a scientific experiment, participants who listened to a single recorded word that was replayed continuously for four minutes routinely heard up to ten slightly different words. Their brains added novelty.

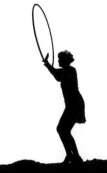

To get out of a rut, create variety. For instance, try to sustain above-head hand hooping while thinking about your whole body. See if something you haven't tried before pops up to dispel boredom. Or confine your hooping to a four-foot square of space, doing as many moves as possible without leaving its boundary. You can limit your workout to on-body, or if you usually hoop on-body, stick to off-body for a session.

Surprises. Make a compilation of fragments of songs with silent spaces in between to listen to while you hoop. Every time the music pauses, stop the hoop in whatever position it happens to be, and do something unexpected. If you are weaving a figure eight and would normally jump through, toss instead, or pass the hoop around your body—anything but what you intended.

Unconventional postures. Try holding a yoga "tree" pose, with one foot raised to the standing leg that is pulsing back and forth to keep the hoop

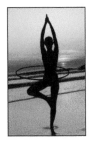

going. Or go against the physics of the hoop. For instance, in shoulder hooping, the chest is normally open as the hoop touches in front, and closed with a rounded back when it touches behind. There is a different quality in maintaining either a closed or an open posture throughout. Likewise, learning to knee hoop, you usually keep the knees together, rotating in the direction the hoop is going. As you develop a stronger relationship with the hoop, you can challenge that basic stance with the knees further apart. That prepares you for stepping and tapping or moving around freely while the hoop hovers above your knees.

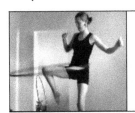

SaFire's Hoopie award-winning video, *Love the Process,* reveals the ways in which experimenting, persisting, and stretching limits pays off.[18] [V]

In summary, to achieve grace with both abandon and discipline, mix it up. Alternate between surprising quickness and fluid slowness. Play with changes in direction, level, and the orientation of your body while doing any familiar move. Do whatever it takes to keep you engaged.

Chapter Three Links

www.HoopDanceBook.com/chapter3

1. *How to Hula Hoop for Beginners: Lift up from Waist to Lasso above Head.* Jul. 10, 2010.

2. *Walking While Hooping.* Feb. 7, 2008.

3. *Hoop Convergence 09—Jewels—Sustained Spin.* Jul. 1, 2009.

4. *Cross Isolation Turn Tango Hoop Dance Tutorial Move— LucasHooping.com.* Apr. 10, 2010.

5. *Hoop Girl from SF.* Jun. 23, 2008.

6. *Hoop Tips & Tricks: Outside Isolations with Jocelyn Gordon.* Mar. 2, 2012.

7. *Pink Moon.* Jul. 3, 2009.

8. *Hoop Dance Tutorial: Anti-Spin Flowers and Sacred Geometry with Rainbow Michael.* Jun. 14, 2011.

9. *Head Hooping 'N Currents.* Oct. 27, 2011.

10. *Shanghai Restoration Project Hoopdance.* Apr. 10, 2010

11. *Brecken Rivara's Hoop Demo.* Feb. 13, 2011.

12. *Hooping—Eye of the Storm.* Nov. 17, 2007.

13. *Hoopalicious—"The Barrel Roll" Tutorial.* Aug. 26, 2008.

14. *Forward Fig 8 Vertical Jump Hoop Tutorial—Hooping Mad.* Apr. 27, 2010.

15. *Symphony of Science—We Are All Connected.* Jan. 9, 2010.

16. *Hoop Poi Tutorial: 5 Beat Weave / Elbow Funk (Without Throws).* Aug. 19, 2010.

17. *World Hoop Day 2011, Brighton, Flash Mob 2.* Nov. 12, 2011.

18. *"Love the Process"—SaFire's Hooping Manifesto (Song: Taio Cruz— I Can Be).* Oct. 15, 2009.

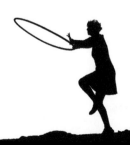

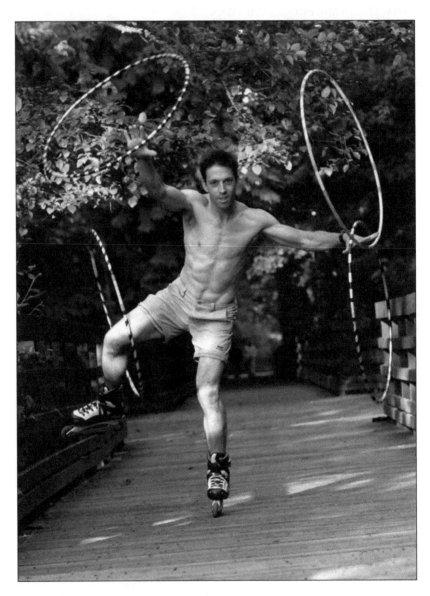

Dizzy Hips hooping on Rollerblades

FOUR

Moving Body, Mind, and Spirit

Everything about you depends on circulation.
—Jack LaLanne, fitness expert and bodybuilder

In our increasingly sedentary world, office workers often have stressful jobs, children spend more time sitting at computers, and even college students may not be getting the level of physical fitness they need. Games help us stay active, but competition often rewards the strong and lowers the self-esteem of less aggressive players. On the other hand, hooping is an affordable and adjustable exercise that's fun and has a fairly level playing field. It provides a healthy workout for people who want to engage their physicality, enhance muscle tone, or develop poise. Adding rhythm-feedback to total-immersion dance, hoopdance works to unify mental, emotional, and physical energy.

Hoop maker Laurie Hobbs learns about life from hoopdance. She says, "I have noticed that the body wants to move with the least effort possible, like water flowing to the lowest point of gravity." Based on that observation, she suggests that we get out of our own way in order to let our motion "come about." As we get better at focusing our intentions, our bodies learn how to meet the hoop in the easiest, most gentle way. "If we allow it," Laurie says, "the mind and spirit will test limits and take the body along for the ride."

Whether we hoopdance for our own physical and emotional health, as a means of expression, or to teach others, there are three components of hoopdance: you, the hoop, and the environment. You manipulate the

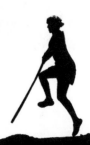

hoop in reaction to dynamic rhythms that may be the sounds you are listening to, remembering, or have stored in your bones. The hoop gains its own momentum, creating a feedback loop of sensory information going to your nerve endings, as you interact with it and it touches your body. All of this happens in an environment, be it your living room, a park, a classroom, or a stage—in solitude or with others.

Mental and Emotional Health

Hoopdance is naturally aerobic and puts no harmful stress on the body when performed correctly. It improves spatial cognition as you learn to anticipate where the hoop is likely to be. And it takes less energy as you gain control and master technique. For maximum benefit you have to challenge yourself the right amount compared to your skills. That means you will eventually develop more complex moves, use smaller hoops, or work on deeper levels of the impediments to flow that may come up in your practice. In return, hooping strengthens your cardiovascular system and metabolism. It also keeps you in a state of active learning, an important factor for maintaining brain health.

Until you master it, simply passing the hoop around your body with your hands can be a brainteaser. Being able to keep both palms downward or upward on the hoop at all times, using a light grip, is not automatic for everyone. At the levels of your waist or knees, hold the hoop out in front of you like a flat disk, with both palms downward on top of the hoop. Let go with one hand to pass the hoop behind you with the other, keeping it on an even horizontal plane. Without seeing where it is, you must grasp the hoop behind with the first hand—palm down. When you let go with the second hand, the hoop comes around to front and you touch it again the way you started. At neck level, palms have to be under the hoop at all times, facing up, and the hoop is kept horizontal without going above the head. If that's too easy, try swinging two hoops in figure-eight patterns, one in front of you, and the other in reverse behind.

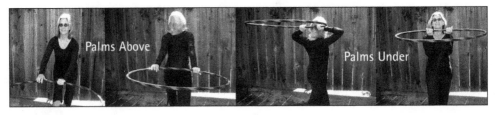

Palms Above

Palms Under

Sharna Rose says, "When the hoop is going around you, you are replicating the three-dimensional molecular dance of reality, connecting with the spin of all existence." Advanced hoopers like Sharna are aware that they use every molecule in their bodies to move the hoop, dip a shoulder, or take a step. The breath pulling in and pushing out controls the expansion and contraction of movement. Effort followed by rest and resistance gives way to yielding and creates contrast.

Mona Qaddoumi (ShpongledHoops) used the universal concept of spinning as a part of her senior thesis in a studio art program at the University of Vermont. Her body and her hoop created a spinning visual artwork, blindfolded in relief against a sketched canvas. The lessons of hoopdance guide her. "While hooping I am conscious of the ebb and flow of each day, of an all-encompassing rhythm, and of my body and the potential usefulness of the empty space surrounding it."[1] [V]

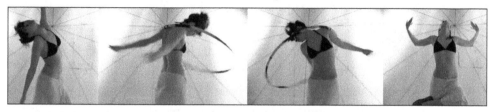

Some scientists believe that consciousness is spread through the fascia, a body-wide system of collagen and elastin fibers that runs from head to toe without interruption. Dana Fonté, a myofascial release therapist in California, says, "The connective tissue of fascia covers and interpenetrates every muscle, bone, nerve, blood vessel, and organ—including the brain and spinal cord—down to the cellular level. If every other part of the body were removed and only the fascia remained, the body would retain its recognizable form."

As we hoopdance, we discover the intelligence that resides not only in our brains but in our bodies as well. We keep the fascia supple, releasing physical tension to unpinch nerves and facilitate the flow of consciousness. As flow calms the mind and energizes the body, intelligence is freed up to deal with uncomfortable emotions that are often magnified in the

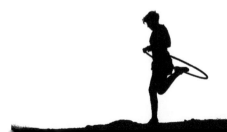

process. Once recognized, these sensations can be transformed. Nayeli Michelle Bouvier, founder of HoopNectar, says she has two secret weapons for inventing beautiful hoopdance moves: "One is my music player headphones that fit around the back of my head, and the other is plenty of emotion to process."

Dispelling Depression

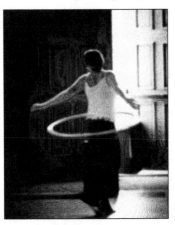

Renee Kogler founded Cleveland Hoop Dance, after hooping alone for hours every day helped her through an identity crisis. Both her parents had died, and she had been separated from her twin sister through marriage. These were the people she depended on to love her most. Their loss cast her into an emotional darkness. "Hooping was like a drug I needed, an antidepressant. It was the only thing I had that made me believe I could love myself, and be beautiful, without needing anyone else to say it." (Renee is profiled in chapter 5)

Jonathan Baxter founded the HoopPath after his depression gradually receded while hooping to exercise an injured shoulder. He says, "It's as if hooping built up my emotional white-blood-cell count. I have more immunity to the disease of depression and more strength to fight it if it creeps in." As his body became more supple and stronger, his view of life changed from feeling cursed to feeling blessed.

When I met traveling nurse Kacey Douglas of Homespun Hoops in Charleston, South Carolina, she was pleased with her life choices. Even so, in her nursing profession she is often faced with unhappy situations that can be draining. The feedback she gets from performing with, selling, and giving away hoops creates an uplifting balance in her life. When she moved to Florida temporarily, her new neighbor, Abby Albaum, helped her make hoops for the company Nomadic State of Mind.

For Abby, hoop obsession replaced depression. Teaching hoopdance and going to hoop jams kept her engaged with life and her feelings. She founded Hoola Monsters in St. Petersburg, Florida.

Teaching Little Hoopers

Hula hooping is play, but hoopdance teachers are reinventing the game for children. Bunny Star and the teachers who work with her in Sydney, Australia, bring larger hoops than are found in the school's equipment locker to an after-school care program. Their young students appreciate getting personal instruction and learning advanced tricks. Bunny says, "We do it so the kids can enjoy moving at the end of the day instead of sitting on couches eating sugar."

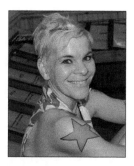

Bunny gets a kick out of seeing children four and five years old get the hoop up on their chests and do other moves that can take adults years to master. "Tapping into that potential early gives kids a tool for sustaining their own happiness. Hoopdance gives them a way to shift their energy when it falls out of balance." She created a television series to use hoopdance to empower children; her *Hoopy Time Show* stars Bunny Hoop Star and the Hoopy Time Heroes. It takes place on a world that needs rescuing when the massive hoop powering it stops spinning. The heroes fly to Earth and pick up a child to help heal Planet Hoolio.[2] V

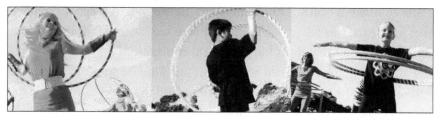

Dizzy Hips

Unlike Hoopy Time's heroes, kids can be easily discouraged trying to develop skills that are difficult to accomplish. Performer and teacher Paul Blair (Dizzy Hips) says, "You can pretty much play with the hoop immediately, so the learning curve can be shallow for a long time, unless you want to make it steep." He encourages kids to experiment. "The hoop is a circle. That's all you have to know. After that you can figure out that it

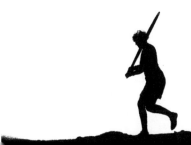

rolls, spins, wobbles, flip-flops, or can balance to stay in one place. You can get inside it, or you can run and push it." He demonstrates by push-

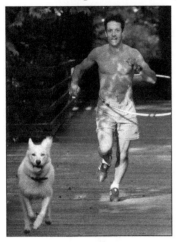

ing a big hoop down the road with another hoop. Then he runs back and forth *through* the big hoop while waist hooping. He also has a 75-pound tractor tire that he hoops with, jumps on, rolls on, and lets roll over him. "Once I find something that gets kids engaged, I keep doing it."

As a child Paul had plenty of time to experiment under his own aegis. He spent most of his time with a German shepherd named Sigi. The gentle dog had been military trained, could climb ladders, and was trusted by Paul's mom more than a human babysitter. During the summers Paul took Sigi to his grandmother's house in Waha, Idaho, where they had freedom to roam the woods.

In school Paul spent most of his time on the "girls' side" of the playground, with jump ropes and hoops or playing on the monkey bars. He often set goals for himself like deciding to throw a ball against a set of stairs to make it bounce once and then hit the fourth stair. "I could do that for hours. Put me in a room for a piano lesson, and it didn't happen. I prefer activities that don't have practical application."

Paul likes going for world records. At age nine he sunk fifty-one basketballs in a row to beat his own record for the most free throws. He has been in *Ripley's Believe It or Not!* and *Guinness World Records*. He created a project to build the world's largest kite, to use as a hang glider, and engaged schoolchildren to help. He gave hoops to schools in exchange for the shiny potato chip bags that come with the children's lunches, and used the tough plastic from the bags to make his kite.

The key to Paul's success as a hoop champion is passion, practice, and focus. He teaches hooping to kids as an example of the ways in which they can learn to use any tool creatively. "Playing provides a place to figure things out, like which techniques can be used to advantage in each game. Look at all the tricks people use in soccer, and all the other games you can play with a soccer ball. It's the same with hooping. These sports allow you to be creative." As movement disciplines are becoming more respected, he says, "activities like hula hooping will be seen as legitimate creative sport." His trick called "hoop spanking" is something I had never thought to do. Tossing a hoop into the air, he paddles it with both hands to keep it aloft.[3] [V]

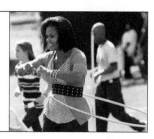

Hooping at the White House, First Lady Michelle Obama challenged schools to provide healthier meals and to allot more time to physical activity.[4] [V]

The Vegetable Circus

When I hitched a ride to the Harbin Hoop Jam in 2010, I met Zach Fischer and Marria Grace (pronounced "MAHria"). They are known as Number Nine and Madame Spinach in the Vegetable Circus, a physical program for kids. Zach met Marria in Boston, where she had been a founding member of the Boston Hoop Troop in 2003. Zach also happened upon a juggler called Hot Soup, and his buddy Gazpacho. They were teaching kids to juggle with oranges at a fair while telling them how good oranges are for their health. When Hot Soup and Gazpacho formed Vegetable Circus, they recruited Number Nine and Madame Spinach to teach an after-school program, complete with hooping and tumbling.

When Marria teaches hooping, beginner park core, or juggling with food, she uses storytelling to bring out the creative silliness in children. For a hoop class she shows up in mismatched brightly colored socks that clash with her purple ruffled pants and orange tank top. "Let's warm up!" she begins, and soon the class is rolling on the floor with hoops. Zach is following along demurely, looking circumspect in his black street pants and muscle shirt, but striped socks of pink on one foot and green on the other are a clue that he might cause some monkey business. Sure enough

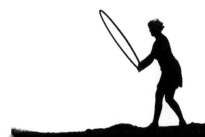

he chimes in to put an anti-spin on the windmill arm-stretching exercise, which has the kids flailing in circles and laughing.

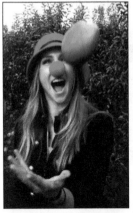

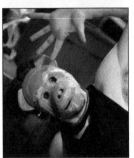

Together Zach and Marria accent instruction with clowning around. They burst into acrobatic hooping, with runs and jumps that stop short in static poses. When Number Nine lifts Madame Spinach into the air, the question arises, "Can we get a hoop up there?" and they do.[5] [V]

Children love to see adults playing with food. Some kids don't see fresh vegetables until they go to college, join the military, or enter the workforce. Vegetable Circus puts whole foods into kids' hands so they can see what it looks and smells like. They can toss a banana into the air and learn that if it gets stepped on, it will go squish. When they play with an orange for twenty minutes and drop it repeatedly, it softens up. Then it's easier to peel, tastes great, and gives them energy. Zach says, "Adding fruits and vegetables to a juggling act is a great way to motivate kids, and they learn that what they put into their bodies affects what they can do—if they don't have proper nutrition, their handstands won't be as good. It gets the kids' attention and gets them moving."

For some kids merely the expectation that they have to move in a certain way makes them freeze up. This is especially true in middle school, when youngsters are often self-conscious and unsure of themselves. At Vegetable Circus no one has to try out for a team or compete against anyone else. Zach says, "Mainstream sports often take place in a competitive atmosphere. We teach kids that they can just move. Everyone can hoop, throw balls, or do handstands any way they want."

Imagine a Vegetable Circus in your city, bringing children access to nutritional information in a way that's fun. Young people learn to control their energy input and output, and when parents get involved, relationships with their children are strengthened.

Hoop Power

At thirty-four years old, social worker Kaye Anderson tried hooping with her twin daughters at a school fundraiser. That was in 2008, and they had so much fun together that Kaye signed up for classes and soon became a certified hoop teacher. "Especially at school, children need to be taught to use the tools adults take for granted. When I taught hooping at my daughters' school as a volunteer, children who otherwise didn't know what to do with themselves on the playground joined in and started interacting with each other."

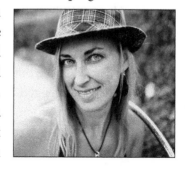

Kaye uses hooping in her clinical practice. Similar to the playground activity of swinging, in which children work to propel themselves through the air, hooping gives her young clients both an adrenaline surge and an emotional release. She finds that hooping calms overstimulated children while creating a space in which they feel safe. That helps some kids to open up and talk more freely.

In the hooping classes Kaye teaches to groups of children, some kids just want to see who can keep the hoop up longest. If they also know many hooping tricks, they dominate the group, clamoring, "Look at me; look what I can do; see how good I am." Her job is to get children to feel confident enough about their own abilities so that they can learn and share together with their peers.

To counter bullying and cliques, Kaye devised a physical puzzle. Her challenge to an entire class is this: figure out how to get everyone all together inside one hoop. Her group of fourth graders wasn't sure she was serious at first. They went through twenty minutes of trying things like getting on each other's shoulders, which included pushing and shoving. Then they went through various stages of grief, until they found a way to include everybody. A class of thirty students came up with the solution that if each child just put one hand in, they could make it work. Then they

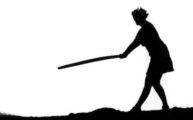

talked about the process: what it felt like to be the one who got left out or the one who got into the hoop and took up all the space.

Group dynamics change over time during Kaye's three-week work-shops. With a group of twenty-seven girls from fourth and fifth grades, she started by giving them plain black hoops in different sizes. Every child tried all the hoops in a game called Freeze Hoop, which is modeled on Musical Chairs but without eliminating anyone. "At the end of that session, each child tagged a hoop as her own, and we talked about what this new toy meant to them."

During the second week the hoops were decorated. At the end of the first hour all the girls had taped their hoops with the three colors of electrical tape that each had chosen. Kaye says, "Taping is not easy, and the girls who finished first stepped in to help others. They were proud that they had made a tangible object and had learned how to use it. They were eager to talk about what worked well and what didn't."

In the third and final week, Kaye teaches hoop tricks. On the last day, only half of the girls were in the group picture. The rest were having too much fun to stop hooping. Kaye will do the same for a group of boys who have protested, "Why do the girls get to hoop? It doesn't have to be a girl thing," which is true.

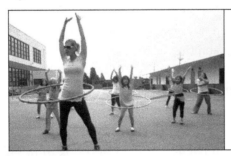

Kaye Anderson's Albany YMCA class was her first-ever Kids Hoop Camp.[6] V

The memory of hooping as a child enhances the experience of hooping as an adult. In proportion to one's size, a big hoop makes adults feel like masterful kids again. That fosters a sense of play. Kaye loves to see self-doubt wash away when an adult she teaches does something that seemed impossible on a playground years ago. When adults learn hooping with children, it gives them an experience to replicate in other situations at other times. Using the hoop as a metaphor for creating boundaries, Kaye says, "Things you can control in your life can be taken inside your hoop. What remains outside of your hoop? There is plenty of material there."

Beginner's Mind

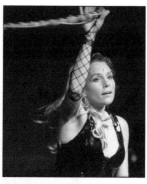

For children with learning difficulties, life often feels like a succession of failures with everyone watching. Learning specialist Heather Toles teaches hooping to special-needs children and to the teachers who teach them. "Learning to hoop helps educators remember viscerally what it is like to try something new. It puts them into beginner's mind, replicating what we ask students to do every day: put yourself out in front of your peers and be okay making mistakes." Heather finds that when her younger students take "brain breaks" from cognitive lessons, they like to play with the hoop. It uses up their excess energy while grounding them in the here and now.

When Heather was a child, not being able to hoop caused her a great deal of frustration and shame. As a woman, hoopdance performance gives her a safe way to express herself in public. "It helped me let go of self-judgment. The hurdle was to understand that if an audience doesn't like what they see in my performance, that's okay; they don't have to watch." Having overcome her own discomfort, she influences others to find courage or solace via the ripple effect. She relates hoopdance to many of life's challenges. "If you drop the hoop, you have a choice: you can pick it up or walk away. To get to flow, you go through bumbling, frustrating, and sometimes embarrassing stages of things not fitting right. But in the end hooping is something everyone can be successful at if they are willing to put in the time."

Ambassadors for Nonviolence

Once Tisha Marina learned to hoopdance, she found it was a great tool for working with youth in the poorer neighborhoods of Los Angeles. "When it gets dark and the gangs come out, so do the drugs. If the children are at

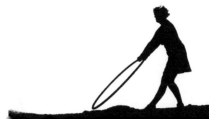

home hula hooping, that gives me joy." Through Safe School Ambassadors she goes to middle and high schools to teach skills that stop bullying. "The trainings I do are intense because I'm teaching nonviolence to violent kids who don't want to listen. Often I have a tough crowd of boys and girls."

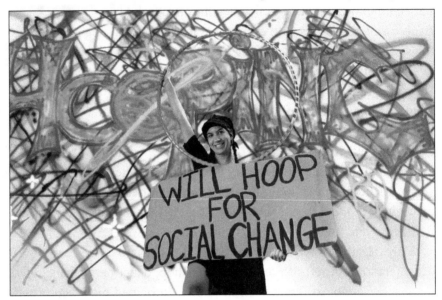

During a particularly difficult training, Tisha laid out twelve of her handmade hoops on the playground at lunchtime and watched. Kids who had been fighting in the classroom rolled the hoops back and forth to each other. She saw them play together. "For a while hardened adolescents became children again. When they came back to the table, they put their shells back on; they had no idea what I had witnessed. They had been free. Those are the moments I live for." She understands that the happiness and freedom experienced by the students in those moments will resurface in the right conditions later on.

In Alabama Dana Moore and Brandy Hughes have a mission similar to Tisha's. They offer a hoopdance ministry as a joint project of AuraHoops and the Dream Center of their local church. They give away hoops that have been prayed over and anointed in oil. Dana says, "The kids have many stresses in their lives. They worry about where they're going to get meals and clothing, and we want to keep them off the streets. If we give them a hoop and they fall in love with it, then they have something to be happy about that keeps them busy in a positive activity."

Four Rhythms for Mind and Body

Betty Shurin (Betty Hoops) discovered hoopdance at a music festival in the mid-1990s. On the day after 9/11, she decided to take the healing

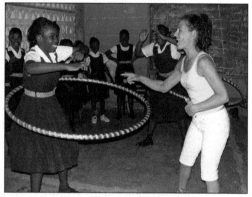

power of hooping to New York City. "That was the place people needed laughter and connection to the earth the most. After ten days of freaking out because there was literally a bomb threat on every bridge that I needed to drive across, I arrived, unpacked my duffel, and got to work." She offered free workshops at dance studios, in Central Park, around Times Square, and in Brooklyn. She hooped with firefighters and police officers who had lost children, inner-city kids who had lost parents, and middle-aged people who had lost faith. People on Wall Street tried the hoops slung over her shoulder, and construction workers came down from scaffolding to give it a try.

In Aspen, Colorado, and in other places throughout the world, Betty teaches children to be hoop warriors with her four-rhythms technique. She gives larger hoops to heavier, taller, and more muscular children and lighter ones to the smaller children. Then she identifies and corrects the five most common mistakes her students make while hooping: looking down, twisting the knees, twisting the torso, moving too slowly, and rolling the hips in a circle.

Once everybody's got the hang of waist hooping, they try three stances that Betty calls "regular" (left foot forward), "neutral" (feet at hip distance apart, side by side), and "goofy" (right foot forward). Next the children hoop while squatting, running in place, and turning in circles to warm

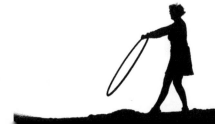

up. Then they hoop to the following four rhythms, each explored with different music.

EARTH: With African drumming music playing, the kids stomp their feet, squeeze their fists, and "grrrr" like a bear. Betty talks about being creative in the circle of their hoop, stomping out their space on the ground, and developing strength, body awareness, balance, and a sense of importance.

WATER: With Caribbean music playing, arms are used to swim like fishes. Kids get to show off their backstroke or nosedive while keeping the hoop spinning and Betty asks them to move like jellyfish, gliding legs across the floor, and then reaching out from their spines as if they have tentacles. When the hoops fall she talks about letting go and understanding that we cannot control everything in life.

FIRE: With tribal and pop music blasting through the room, it is time to dance with attitude. "Use your body to show your strength. There is no wrong way to move, just keep moving and breathing!" The kids harness their power by stopping abruptly, while the hoop keeps spinning. After thirty seconds of standing still they spin with renewed energy. In this segment Betty fosters enthusiasm, creativity, and a sense of individuality.

AIR: With quieter, easy listening music to guide their breathing, students open their arms as they inhale, pushing hands out in front as they exhale. They become eagles soaring through the sky, weightlessly surveying land and sea. Breath is used to keep them afloat and calm, aware of what is in their minds and what is going on around them.

Then, in silence, Betty asks her students to slow down their breathing, relinquish thoughts, and stand in place with arms outstretched in resting pose. She observes, "At assemblies of over a hundred kids there is plenty of external stimuli, yet 99 percent of them close their eyes and get deeply into this."

Performing at the end of each class is optional. While peers and teachers clap to the music, students get to choose whether or not they want to enter the circle to show off what they have learned. If they do, Betty encourages them to be silly and have fun. There is no competition, only encouragement. With large groups of children outside of class, Betty demonstrates tricks or creates "teams" to run while hooping from one end of a room or field to the other.

Minding Body and Soul

Many of the teachers I learned from offer teacher-training courses. I took Betty's weekend version, with three other novitiates, and am certified to teach her beginning hoopdance program. After her years of coaching and studying thousands of bodies in motion, Betty identifies poor alignment or body mechanics as the most common obstruction to healthy hooping. Throughout the weekend, she taught us to correct our own carriage and to recognize, in others, the five most common restrictions for adults as they learn to hoopdance.

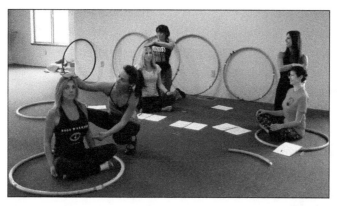

- An S curve in the spine creates compression in the lower back and shoulder blades.
- Hyperextension of the head, or jutting out the chin, creates compression between the shoulder blades.
- Hyperextening the knees forces the knees back beyond their normal straightened position, creating compression in the lower back.
- Sinking into either hip shifts balance and grinds into the hip joint.
- Sinking into the gut creates poor organ function and limits breathing.

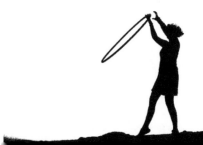

Betty says, "When the body stores pain, it loses power, and we feel depleted. The deep exhaling and inhaling that occurs while hooping replenishes vital energy. Whether you want to flatten your tummy or find inner peace so that you can love your tummy the way that it is, hooping can get you there." Her program embraces both the spiritual and the sports aspects of hoopdance. She leads yoga and hooping retreats, holds Guinness World Records for hooping distance and speed, and hoops while snowboarding.[7] Ⅴ

Hooping through Pregnancy

In 1969 I practiced yoga to prepare for the birth of my first child. In more recent years, many women have safely hoopdanced through their pregnancies, modifying exertion with self-awareness and larger, lighter hoops.

By letting the hoop ride above or below the pregnant belly and using off-body moves, expectant moms can maintain a normal level of activity during pregnancy, often helping to balance erratic moods and sometimes resulting in shortened labor. If you are pregnant and want to hoopdance, follow your care practitioner's advice.

If you are healthy, hooping may benefit your birthing process by keeping you centered and relaxed during gestation, and making you stronger and more flexible for birth. Postpartum hooping can help new mothers regain equilibrium, abdominal strength, and general fitness.

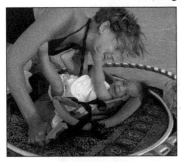
Bonnie MacDougall experienced a short postpartum depression after the birth of her first son, Wynter. She loved to hoopdance but hesitated to take a class, not quite believing she would still be able to do it, yet believing that she needed to be there. At the end of her first class she was crying tears of relief, remembering that she was more than a mom. "I am an adult and a hooper, and here was a whole community of people just like me." She went on to become a HoopPath teacher and hooped all the way through her second pregnancy.

Learning specialist Heather Toles hooped through the last trimester of her first pregnancy after almost four months of mandatory bed rest. "I hula hooped in the hospital to get labor going, and my daughter was born healthy and strong."[8] [V]

Hoopnotica's Preg-O Tools

Rayna McInturf saw her Hoopnotica business partner, Gabriella Redding, hoopdance through pregnancy and then used her own hooping experience to develop a safe system for other pregnant women. It includes a lighter weight Preg-O hoop and a fourteen-page e-booklet that gives advice for modifying a beginner level of hooping throughout the trimesters of pregnancy.

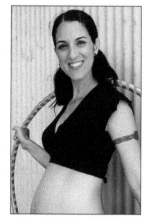

Though morning sickness threatened to keep Rayna at home, she did not give up teaching when she was pregnant. Even if she had nausea, it went away as soon as she started to hoopdance, About safety she says, "There are many layers between the hoop and the baby: muscles, fat, uterus, and amniotic fluid. The baby is completely protected and cushioned even when you hoop around the waist. Remember to keep your heart rate within a safe range, and enjoy yourself." Rayna's prenatal hooping performance proves the point beautifully.[9] [V]

Get Happy and Sweaty

Pregnancy aside, hoopdance has a remarkable way of sculpting and reshaping the body in all the right places. Maneuvering the hoop requires constant push-pull contractions in your core muscles, buttocks, arms, and thighs. In a University of Wisconsin-La Crosse study, sixteen women ranging in age from sixteen to fifty-nine regularly attended choreographed hooping classes. Their oxygen consumption, heart rate, and physical exertion were measured over the course of the study. The average heart rate was 151 beats per minute, and they burned an average of 210 calories in each thirty-minute workout.

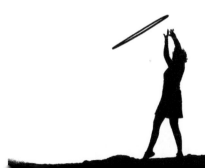

Hoopdance teaches us to properly use muscles, it improves alignment, and burns calories. Still, weight-loss expectations can sometimes be distorted as hoopdance filters into the mainstream fitness industry. When students called Anah Reichenbach to say that hooping in front of the TV fifteen minutes a day for two weeks hadn't resulted in weight loss, she offered three reasons for their disappointment:

- Turn off the TV and engage with the joy of movement. You need excitement to lose weight.

- If you are hooping because you feel fat, your negative self-image will slow your metabolism.

- There is no such thing as easy weight loss. You have to get happy *and* sweaty.

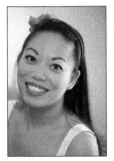

Natasha Young (Hoopsie Daisy), Isopop's Rich Porter, and Julie Schoolastra (Hooptopia) are perfect examples of how hoopdance moves us toward optimal body weight.

Natasha has a full figure and doesn't measure her health with numbers. "How you feel and how your clothes fit are more important than what you weigh. When I was younger, I was so skinny that people were constantly making me eat something. In college I put on the typical 'freshman fifteen.' Having the extra weight made me feel healthy at exactly one hundred and ten pounds."

For almost a decade, living in Southern California where it was sunny most of the year, Natasha walked a lot and didn't have to go to a gym for exercise. But after college she moved to Berkeley, where she knew almost no one, and then 9/11 happened. The slightly cooler climate, combined with her naturally slowing metabolism, her mild depression about the circumstances of her own situation, and the news of world events made her feel lazy. Her weight crept up to one hundred and forty pounds before she realized it was happening. She needed serious exercise.

Natasha bought a mini-trampoline and tried listening to music or watching TV while bouncing, but it didn't last. It wasn't until she rediscovered the fun she used to have in college dance classes that she became fully engaged with hooping. "I huffed and puffed and sweat like crazy! I could feel the difference in just a few months—in my attitude and in my body. Most importantly, you could see how much happier I looked—all from hooping with friends for an hour once a week." By 2009 she was performing in San Francisco clubs and in the city's Flow Show.[10] Ⓥ

Rich had a similar experience. He was physically inactive for six years after high school. Exercise was hard for him. "I had a sedentary lifestyle in college, and then a nine-to-five job working less than a mile from my home. Walking to the office and back was the only exercise I got. By doing something that was not *for* exercise but that actually *is* exercise, I began to have fun moving my body again. Even the way I walk down the street has changed." By hooping and not drinking alcohol, he lost over fifty pounds.

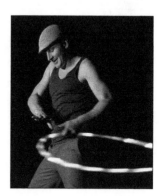

Julie teaches, performs, and hoops for the fun of it in Las Vegas, Nevada, but she was a closet hooper when she started out. She taught herself to hoopdance in her backyard, with only her dog as witness. She was not a natural; everything she learned to do took countless hours of sweat and sometime, even tears, but she kept at it. She lost sixty pounds, improved her posture, and gained self-assurance.

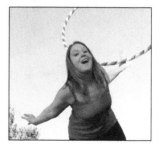

Closing the Circle

Actress Sandi Schultz (Sass) shares the healing power of hoopdance with women in South Africa because of the high rates of rape and child molestation there. "I want others to experience that window of opportunity in which they can forget about everything, without realizing what's

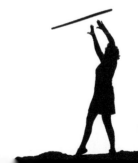

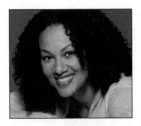

happening, and find a way to be whole again. The relevance of my being a rape and incest survivor is that I can tell other women, 'I've been there and got through it. You can get through it too.' The hoop had a crucial role to play in my story; sharing that is the biggest healer." She began by holding workshops at a school for disadvantaged girls, and guiding women in hooping after speaking engagements. "It was scary how many of them pulled me aside and whispered, 'Thank you for your story; it happened to me too.' Hooping may seem frivolous, but there is immense opportunity for growth beneath its guise of having fun." Her hoopdance workshops help women experience the joy of full-bodied movement.[11] [V]

Sass's story of being victimized by boys and men was sobering to hear. She was just four years old when her cousins held her down and rubbed

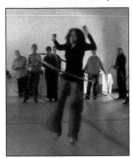

up against her in a pantry, warning her not to tell. At nine, an uncle promised her five cents if she would open her mouth when he kissed her good night. She was in the principal's office at twelve, when the career counselor nonchalantly stepped behind her and slid both his hands over her breasts, beneath her shirt, saying she was "smart enough to be a doctor." Then came the dirty-old-man piano teacher who forever made her toss aside any aspirations for music. "My mother never could understand why. It was another secret to add to the 'Big Secret' I was already spending all my energy guarding. No one was as awful as my stepfather when he got me alone." Now she is grateful to the many wonderful men in her life who have proven that all men are not monsters.

Sass's Message: If you're a survivor, report what happened,
find someone safe and trusted to speak to,
carry your head high, and realize it's not your fault.
YOU CAN SURVIVE THIS.
If you're someone who wants to help, there are many
organizations working with survivors.
Donate your time and money on the Rape Crisis website.
www.rapecrisis.org/rape_how_to_help.html

Being raped as an adult in her Johannesburg home was the last straw for Sass. Six months later she walked away from her homeland, career, house, family, and possessions, staying away from all she had known, in an attempt to recover on her own. In Los Angeles she discovered hoopdance. "Hooping gave my inner little girl a chance to play, and the woman in me found a safe way to reactivate my body. When I hoop, I use my hips and lower chakras in a nonsexual way, and it is impossible not to be joyful. Frightening thoughts can't get through when I am mastering something new and am caught up in learning."

> The chakras are a system of energy fields within each person that governs his or her wellness. Each chakra relates to an aspect of consciousness and body function, and to a color.

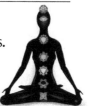

Sass went back to Johannesburg after twelve years in Los Angeles, to accept what she thought would be a temporary role in a television series. The series was renewed for a second season, a third, and a fourth. Then one year at the stroke of midnight on the anniversary of her rape, she was fire hooping in Johannesburg and realized that she had to revisit the house she had abandoned so many years before. The next day a woman who was living in the house let Sass in to hoopdance in an empty room, on the very spot where she had been violated as an adult.

Sass hoopdanced in spirals around the scene of the crime against her. "I dropped to my knees as a vortex of negative energy whooshed through the hoop and away through the floor. It felt as if, after years, I was able to leave unnecessary baggage where it belonged." Her friend captured the dance on video, but the recording does not show what Sass was experiencing. You cannot see, on screen, the moment in which she stopped running, when she turned around and said "boo," to the demons she had been living with and fearing for so long.

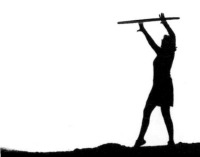

Chapter Four Links

www.HoopDanceBook.com/chapter4

1. *Performance Hoop Dance: Crumblenaut.* Mar. 25, 2009.

2. *Hoopy Time Teaser.* Aug. 31, 2010.

3. *Hoop Spanking with Dizzy Hips.* Apr. 2, 2011.

4. *First Lady Michelle Obama Hula Hoop at Whitehouse.* Oct. 22, 2009.

5. *Ninja Hoops at Athletic Playground.* Dec. 4, 2011.

6. *Hoop-Dance Class with Kaye Anderson.* Sep. 8, 2011.

7. *Extreme Hula Hooping on a Snowboard—Betty Hoops.* May 17, 2010.

8. *Hoopnobirthing3-1-11.MP4.* May 14, 2011.

9. *Hoopnotica Prenatal Hooping Performance at DCAC Fitness Convention.* May 6, 2009.

10. *Natasha at Flow Show—4/24/09.* Apr. 25, 2009.

11. *Sass Women's Workshop July 2007.* Aug. 2, 2008.

PART II

The Revolution

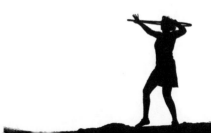

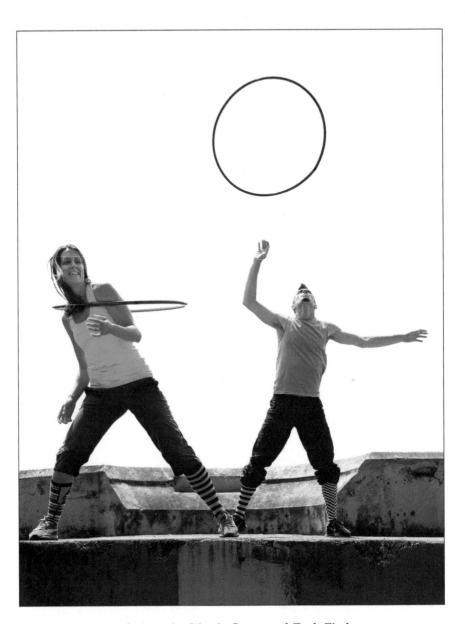

Revolutionaries Marria Grace and Zach Fischer

FIVE

Joining the Revolution

You have to do the thing you're afraid of most
before you get the courage to do it.

—George Clooney, in the movie *Three Kings*

Hoopdance Formentera

Nico Gerbi, an Italian translator living in Spain who splits his time between Barcelona and the small island of Formentera off the city's coast, helped me collect many hoopdance stories. I met him in 2007, just months before my first hoopdance class, while traveling with a friend. Our travel package included a car for sightseeing in Barcelona, and Nico was the driver. We convinced him to take us out of the city, along the coast to the Dalí museum. He showed us a medieval town as well, and we talked about the nature of truth at lunch and coffee stops along the way.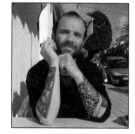
When I visited him the following year, I brought a hoop. He appreciated it as an American icon but hung it on his wall, where it remained unused.

Later, when I was wondering how to meet hoopdancers in other parts of the country, Nico decided to tour the States with a friend from Korea. They planned to drive a big, 1980s American car coast to coast. In the end his friend couldn't make the trip. Instead, Nico agreed to drive through eighteen states, east of the Rocky Mountains, in an economical late-model rental as my research assistant. His participation gave me the courage to spend four weeks on the road. We switchbacked 4,300 miles from New York to New Orleans, interviewing hoopdancers all along the way.

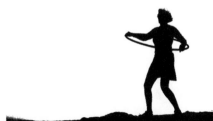

Nico had learned to break dance in 1985. He was living with his family in the center of Italy near Camp Darby, the biggest American army base in Europe, and he was thirteen years old. "A friend of mine had a friend who was an American guy. We started hanging out with him and his friends, spending entire afternoons doing tricks and dancing to their black music." "Nineteen," a song by Paul Hardcastle about America's involvement in the Vietnam War, was his first break-dancing song.[1] M

In break-dance music, James Brown's drumbeats are often sampled, and that led Nico to an interest in funk music. Then slower electronic music allowed him to dance for many hours at a time in clubs and at raves and parties. His overall style became a mix of those influences, eventually getting fast and upbeat again.

When Nico was my research assistant, we took classes with many hoopdancers. In North Carolina he even experienced a "need" to hoop. Yet when he returned to Spain, his own hoop stayed on the wall until August 2010. He finally took it to a beach party. "They couldn't believe I was able to do those little tricks I learned on the road. Now I've been invited to hoop at three more parties. Power to the hoop. Hoopdancing got to Formentera!"

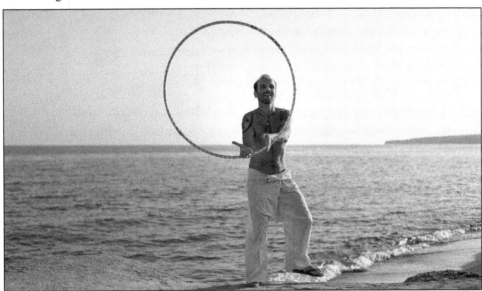

Spindarella

Nico and I had started our trip by interviewing members of Groovehoops in New York. From there I had scheduled a stop in Baltimore, because I wanted to meet Michele Clark, seven of clubs in the deck of The Hooping Life Playing Cards, also a member of Groovehoops, and one of the few African American hoopers I knew of at the time. Unable to reach her in advance, I called from the car. She was in Philadelphia and needed a ride back to Baltimore, so we picked her up.

Nico told Michele he had thought of hoopdancing as a white middle-class sport, and asked what she thought. "It probably started that way," she said, "but the hoop has the potential to cross racial and economic borders. People usually get intro-duced to hooping either through someone they know or at an event where they see it taking place. It just takes this simple human transference method to eventually introduce hooping to everyone." In her own practice Michele emulates break danc-ers, because the form makes room for seemingly impossible new moves to emerge spontaneously. As a teacher she urges people to get out of whatever physical or mental box they have for hoop-dance. "Break apart what is known, get in touch with the hidden parts of yourself, and take risks."

Michele's video channel is called Spin0da0rella, and as a child one of her favorite activities was to twirl around until she fell down laughing. At five years of age she was asked, "What do you want to be when you grow up?" She said, "I want to be a belly dancer." Sensing disapproval of her answer, she announced that she would become a scientist. Everyone was relieved that she might follow in the footsteps of other family members. Even so, she asked her parents for dance classes, and they agreed, but it had to be African dance.

Michele wonders if scientists share the intense feelings of love for other scientists that she has for other hoopdancers.

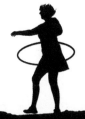

At fifteen Michele found a radio station that hosted *The Grateful Dead Hour* from eleven P.M. until midnight, and then live music until dawn. "It was free-form instrumental that conveyed an ecstatic feeling, and led me to seek out bands that played that type of music. I saw people at the concerts moving freely without concern for the quality of their dancing. It was liberating."

In college Michele studied art. Like science, it engaged her intellect. It wasn't dancing, but she was getting closer to creative expression. Then at a music festival in the Berkshires, she met the people who would go on to form Groovehoops. They were impressed by what she could do with a hoop, and she confessed to having been the hula-hooping champion of her elementary school. She spent the night in their extra tent, and they sent her home with a hoop and an invitation to visit them in New York.

In Baltimore Michele practiced on her rooftop and visited Groovehoops in New York on the weekends. "We were a mobile party on the streets. Malcolm Stuart would beat box, sing, and rap, as we walked around with our hoops and took them on the subway. All but a couple of us were living together at the Happy Robot, a loft in Brooklyn." When she left the group, she hadn't realized there was a larger hoopdance community. In Baltimore she met other hoopers, but none with the skills she had developed with Groovehoops.[2] V

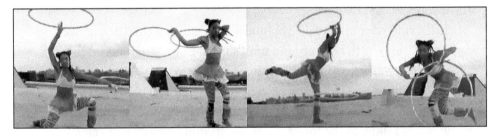

Then Michele saw Brecken Rivara do a behind-the-back, elbow-to-elbow transfer at a college event. "I could see that she knew what she was doing. Anything I showed her she could just do. I gave her my phone number, and she actually called me. Brecken became my best hoop friend in Baltimore. We hooped in the park at least once a week for three years, and she introduced me to hooping videos on the Web."

Michele recalls watching videos of other hoopers. "I got into a sort of hoop-tricks arms race with myself, an internal competition that kept my mind occupied with the unproductive question, 'What crazy thing can I do next?'" She stopped watching videos and began learning yoga to make a deeper physical connection with herself. Then she saw a woman practice the martial art of capoeira. "I couldn't tell at first whether it was dancing or stretching, but I started to understand that all movement disciplines engage us in a process that reveals the way we approach ourselves and others." That insight led her to establish her hoopdance career.

Being Gorgeous

After we dropped Michele off in Baltimore, Nico and I headed inland to the little township of Adams, Pennsylvania, to see Stephanie Babines. We were surprised when she asked Nico to wait in the car while she showed me around her studio. Later we went to a café, and she explained.

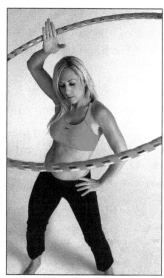

When Stephanie applied for a license to open her Oh My You're Gorgeous dance studio, there was trouble. Because she wanted to teach pole dancing as well as hoopdance, belly dance, and yoga, township officials feared that her business might turn into a place to train strippers. That was the furthest thing from Stephanie's mind. She encourages her students to feel beautiful inside and out, and sexy rather than lewd, as they dance with hats, boas, and high-heeled shoes from her collection of costumes.

Initially barred from teaching her classes, Stephanie was ready to put her house up for sale in order to take her case to federal court. First she went to the ACLU office and filled out a seven-page application. "That same day, they took my case for free on the grounds that my first amendment rights were being violated."

A settlement was reached after Stephanie agreed to have no men in the studio, no nudity, and no unenrolled people watching when classes were in session. She also agreed to turn off her neon sign whenever she left

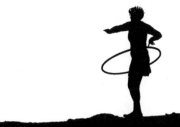

the studio, which makes the parking lot pitch-dark at the end of evening classes, but she was eventually allowed to open her business. The neighbors have never complained. At the nearby bakery, restaurant, and beauty shop, the women who take Stephanie's classes are always welcomed.

Stephanie worked as a computer programmer before hooping helped her to lose two inches from her waistline in a month. "In college I was really heavy and was looking for a way to get fit. On a girls' night out with my friends, someone said I should install a pole in my house because it is a great workout. It was meant as a joke, but I took it seriously." She found a DVD of pole dancing for fitness and called the instructor who made it. After training in Las Vegas she was certified as a pole dance teacher. "I lost weight and strengthened my core, but I still had a little belly. That's where hoopdance came in."

In her studio Stephanie teaches children starting at age four, and her oldest student is eighty-eight years old. In the summer she offers a hoop group every Sunday morning, bringing families together with the idea that they can make time for each other with hoopdance in the big field of a neighborhood park.

Cleveland Hoopdance

Nico and I bid Stephanie good-bye and typed our next destination into the GPS, which led us to a bright yellow farmhouse in Mantua, Ohio, near

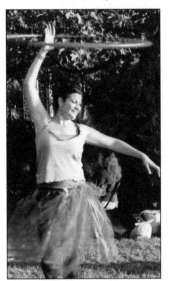

Cleveland. We stayed with Renee Kogler, her husband, David, and their daughter, Willow. We danced in the living room with Willow, Nico played music with David in his studio, and Renee hooped for us in the backyard.[3] V

Renee had grown up on the south side of Chicago with her twin sister, Karen, but in their early twenties Renee's marriage to David separated them. "As kids we were pals, roller-skating and riding our bikes, apart from everyone else. When I got married, learning to be my own person was hard. I expected the same intensity from my life with David that I'd had with Karen." Trying to figure out what her new place in life was, Renee became insecure and melancholic.

She tried belly dancing and took other classes to fill the void inside, but nothing relieved her loss of connection.

It wasn't until she saw photographs of hoopers on Tribe.net that things began to change. "I thought, 'Whatever they have, I need it.' I perceived love and vitality in their photographs. They looked comfortable, settled, and whole, and they had hoops in their hands." Hoops seemed to be making the difference, so Renee and her belly-dancing friends purchased toy hoops and began to play with them.

When Renee saw an adult-sized hoop in the park, she made some like it for herself, her sister, Karen, and their mother, Grace. Then something unexpected happened on June 21, 2007. It was a sunny, summer day. "We were hooping in the yard, listening to Cyndi Lauper. The song 'True Colors' was playing. The lyrics are about being beautiful. When we heard 'Why are you so sad?' we all began to cry without knowing why." It turned out that hooping was Renee and Karen's last connection to Grace. The next day their mother had a massive heart attack and died.

Renee was appointed executor of her mother's estate. "Losing mom ripped the family apart. My dad had passed away six years prior, and Mother was the glue that held us together." Renee wanted to crawl into a hole and never speak to anyone again. She was deeply depressed. When she was alone, hooping in her living room became the only light that penetrated her darkness. It was the only spark of hope she could feel when even the people who loved her most couldn't get through to her.

In that solitude Renee let her body move in ways she had not previously experienced. "Hooping became my prayer, my love, the only thing that connected me to life. In the circular motion I realized that we are all only here temporarily, and in a split second any one of us could be gone." Reaching out from her darkest moments, she found people in the hooping community who helped her actively reengage in life, and then she founded Cleveland Hoop Dance.

Renee's husband, David, is a musician and they support each other creatively. She says, "Hooping and music go together. You *can* have one without the other, but it's much more fun with both. When David's band played

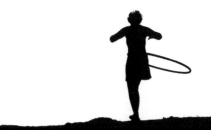

in a festival, I performed with them, and we began to think about creating a vaudeville show together—beyond the living room and the backyard."

Super Hoopers

Next Nico and I drove through the Indiana cornfields and south to Memphis to meet Hooping.org columnist Lara Eastburn, who was beginning her first independent tour to teach hoopdance around the country. She

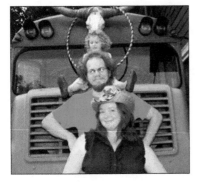

and her family had taken over a vegetable-oil-run 1992 school bus, a renovated RV they had formerly used for trips to Burning Man.

I timed our travel to catch Lara's class in a bar that had an adjacent performance room with a music system. There were hoops everywhere in the spacious black box theater when we arrived, and people were milling about greeting each other as if it were a reunion party. Lara told me,

"The hoopdancers here in Memphis were mostly learning from videos. Many of them knew each other online or by reputation but had never met in person." Before the class began participants were excitedly showing each other moves and trying out each other's hoops.

As a teacher, Lara is captivating; she dances with abandon and exuberance, giving personal attention and encouraging others to take the spotlight. I never would have guessed that there was a time when she would not dream of dancing in public. Previously she had performed as a singer with a blues band. She was singing on an outdoor stage in Baton Rouge, Louisiana, when she saw an enormous black hoop lying to one side. She told herself, "You know what? I'm going to get in that thing. It's a hoop. I won't really be dancing."

The force field inside the hoop felt so good that Lara hoopdanced for twelve hours straight. Then she discovered Hooping.org and instructions for making hoops. "I made some monstrously ugly hoops at first, but every morning I got up and just tried to do something new with them." While she was finishing her doctorate in French literature and teaching at Emory University, she was living with several housemates but never saw anyone else hooping. Then after a year, her housemate Barry picked up the hoop when he thought no one was looking. Lara covertly watched him play with the hoop off-body, something she had not thought to do.

As a shared activity, hooping grew in interest for Lara and Barry. When they saw LED hoops, Barry and another engineer from Georgia Tech came up with an affordable version that they could produce for themselves and sell to others. Hoopdancing had already freed up Lara's sensuality; now it was broadening her whole family's horizons. In 2002 Barry, Lara, and her husband, Drew, established Superhooper.org to sell their hoops. Then Drew quit his day job after Lara gave birth to their daughter, Navi, and the family went on the road. All they needed to make their business mobile was an Internet connection, access to shipping, and their supplies.

Lara and her husband complement each other. Drew doesn't hoop, but he loves to drive. Lara teaches hoopdance everywhere they go. They followed the weather, living in state parks. Lara says, "We can set up a circus tent and work in there with our tools: drilling, soldering, gluing, and grinding. Most parks have electricity." With a cell phone she could still talk to her brother, who was in the air force in Afghanistan.

After the Memphis class, Lara was headed for the heartland. She would bring her hoops to small towns where few people had seen another hoopdancer in person.

Nadia's Dream

Nadia Sophia, our Memphis host, plays with fire: spinning *poi*, eating fire, and hoopdancing with fire wicks on her hoop. She appreciated Lara's mission because the class brought people together. "The best thing about that evening was being around so many hoopers at one time. Everyone had something to share."

Nadia's first dream was to build a library and community center for the village in the Philippines that her mother's family comes from. Through school, she had been to the Dominican Republic on a scholarship the year before we met. She had camped with her class on the beach. Their assignment was to design renovations for buildings and an irrigation system. She believes that fire dancing could have helped her in that situation. "If you

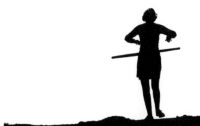

spend creative time with people, you gain their trust. If I were spinning fire when I was in the Dominican Republic I probably would have made more friends and connections, and been able to make my own design better than it was."

When Nadia performed with her drummer friend Mat, he breathed fire into great gusts of flame to get a crowd's attention, and then continued fire breathing behind her fire dancing to enhance the show's overall visual effect. Nadia would like to add comedy to her act, but she says, "So far I'm not very funny or expressive in the way that many of the burlesque hoopdancers are."4 V

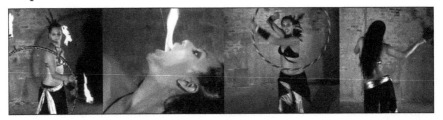

As performing and teaching took over more of Nadia's time in undergraduate school, her focus shifted to movement therapy. She has studied martial arts, music, architecture, art and design, and psychology, and has performed and taught fire arts and hoopdance. Each skill is like a brick in the strong wall of self-knowledge she is building. She brings capoeira and hoopdancing into her graduate dance therapy program at Lesley University in Cambridge, Massachusetts.

Brandy Hoops

After Memphis, Nico and I headed east again. We became a bit lost in Birmingham and arrived in Pell City at the home of Dana and Benjamin Moore after dark. Their family and friends were waiting on a big porch with music and hoops. We visited and played long into the night. Dana's story is included in chapter 11; among her friends we met Brandy Hughes.

Brandy confided that she had been severely overweight and unhappy when she started hoopdancing. She had been practically raised in a gym because her mother had been a basketball coach, and Brandy played sports from childhood through college. "Even so," she says, "I was always a bulky person, not very feminine or happy in my body." After the birth of her first child, she continued to gain weight until she reached 265 pounds. Then she saw her sister's friend hoopdancing. "Dana was doing a crazy style of hula hooping with a bigger hoop than I had ever seen. It took me weeks

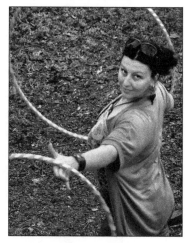

to be able to keep it on my waist for more than a minute, but I wouldn't give up." She accomplished knee hooping first, because it was too hard for her to move her core. (More on knee hooping at the end of this chapter.)

Just from trying hard, and bending over to pick up the hoop every time it fell, Brandy lost two pounds in the first week. That gave her hope and eventually the courage to quit a retail manage-ment job that she hated. "I had never before even imagined being out of work and would always find a new job before leaving an old one. After a few months of hoopdance I decided to stay home with my son Nacoa." She didn't have the financial freedom she wanted, but being at home was what she needed to do for her health and her family.

Hooping in earnest, Brandy lost a 120 pounds in fourteen months, cut-ting out red meat because she realized that it did not agree with the type of energy she needed for hoopdance. "I toned and became aware of my diet. Now if I overeat in a day, I hoop more." What she began as a physical practice was also an emotional tool. She saw that getting up to hoop made her feel stronger and helped her to overcome shyness. "It also made me more graceful and gave me the ability to dance, which I never had before. I got healthier and began to meditate, taking quiet time just for myself. That's really hard to do with young children at home, but hooping gives me a way to quiet down, find my center, and stop worrying."

Brandy's husband, Danny, thought she was crazy at first, but grew to support her all the way. Nacoa loves to tell his friends at school that his mommy hoops. Brandy loves knowing that she brings a healthy lifestyle into her home, which is good for the future of her children.

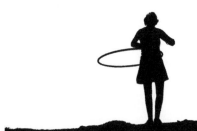

Brandy taught herself some of the moves she didn't learn from Dana, by watching tutorials on the Internet. Then she went to work for Dana's hoopdance company AuraHoops, eventually teaching the weekly classes. She chose "BHoops" as a stage name for performing at health conferences She aims simply "to hoop every day." If she gets in only fifteen minutes, she's happy, and on days when she teaches or offers hoop jams in the park, it's easy to get a good workout.

"Working with AuraHoops comes first," Brandy says, "but doing something on my own is new and fun for me." Volunteering in rural Alabama, Brandy works with autistic children, with women in a shelter, and at a camp for youth with diabetes. Stepping out of her comfort zone and going out to meet new people is empowering. "Showing someone else that they can hoopdance is exciting, so I'm always ready to show the next person." In a video tutorial, she shows us how to duck into a hoop while turning with it stalled on one arm. Placing the hoop on her shoulder, she spins continuously with her arm raised slightly until the hoop lifts to the horizontal plane. Bending her head down and slowing, she lets the hoop overtake her center and then pops right up into it.[5] [V]

Sharing the Pleasure

At the end of our trip Nico and I spent several days in New Orleans and then flew to California. He spent a week at Stinson Beach before returning to Spain, and I went home to Berkeley. Josette Gasse was in town during one of her visits from France to perfect her English. The previous year she had joined me for hooping in the park during her third visit to Berkeley. "The first time I went to the park with Jan," she admits, "I was afraid of ridicule because everyone else seemed at ease with the hoop. But there is a saying in France: *Le plaisir est toujours plus grand lorsqu'il est partagé* (Pleasure increases when it is shared). I had to jump into the water."

After dropping the hoop several times, Josette managed to make a full circle. After an hour she was a fan of hoopdance, and from that moment she became my true hooping friend. She says, "Using two, three, and more hoops at the same time demonstrates that our bodies are just waiting to speak to us if we make a little space, having fun as a child would." She can twirl a hoop in each hand while waist hooping, and she throws herself a little challenge from time to time, but mostly she loves dancing with the hoop. "Sometimes, hooping to fast music, I feel as if I am breathing air from another place and time. To be honest, in the hoop I feel like I am at the center of the world with beneficial waves of energy all around me."

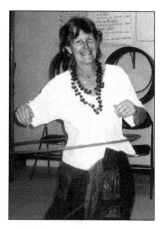

Before Josette started to hoopdance, she had undergone a surgical procedure that limited the use of her left arm. She could do her usual tasks without a problem, but when she tried off-body hooping, she realized how limited her range of motion was. The mobility of her arm came back gradually with persistent gentleness as hooping became part of her regular routine back in France. "After I work hard with my body—painting the walls of my house, digging in the garden, and such—I use my hoop to loosen up and do some stretching."

In the Normandy countryside, Josette's niece attended a therapy retreat to break down her psychological barriers to happiness by shouting, singing, crying, or whatever else it took. Josette gave the younger woman a hoop and told her, "If you have money, you can continue to participate in these seminars to regain your naïveté, or you can hoop, let yourself go in the music, and dance. It is free and just as valuable!" Hooping helped Josette to drop her fear of ridicule, to reengage the right-brain process, and to recall the sweetness of holding hands and singing rounds in a circle at her childhood school.

Midschool Crisis

At the beginning of 2012, Nico had an Internet connection for the first time in his home on the island of Formentera. He sent me an e-mail asking for help with shoulder hooping, and I began searching for a tutorial that got started quickly because his connection to the Web was slow. That's how I found Aaron Smith, a high school senior and one of the finalists for the Youth of the Year Hoopie Award with his E.T. video.[6] V

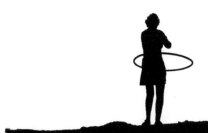

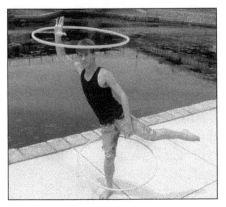

As a sophomore Aaron had a mini midschool crisis. He had lived all his life in Frostburg, Maryland, a small college town in the Appalachian highlands. "It was almost the end of the year," he recalls, "and the seniors were about to graduate. It hit me that I would graduate soon as well. I thought about my senior yearbook. What would I be remembered for?" He was good at running, but that seemed very forgettable.

There had been little for Aaron to do after school, and one day in July 2010 he was watching a video of his favorite band, Blood on the Dance Floor, which led him to discover hoopdance. "Out of nowhere, one of the lead singers came onto stage with an LED dance hoop. I told myself, 'This is it; this is what I need to learn to do.' I knew it was something that would stay in people's minds." He ordered a hoop and began learning by himself. A year later he saw a tutorial by a woman who lived ten miles away, and he found the courage to be a leader. He contacted her on Facebook, and they organized a workshop and jam. "Today there is a hoop community in the area where I live, and I put a lot of work into planning hoop jams that are free for everyone."

At first, Aaron didn't want his parents or anyone else to see him practice, fearing their disapproval. Then he won a talent show. It was his "coming out" with fire and hoops. Only his closest friends had been privy to the new activity before he shared it in three performances. One was for the school's freshmen and sophomores, another for juniors and seniors, and then a show for parents in the evening. Instantly he went from being a normal kid who felt lost in the crowd to one who stood out with pride. Teachers he had known for years congratulated him in amazement. The judges declared him "winner" at the final performance, and his trophy was awarded at the academic pep rally in front of the entire school.

Next came the title of "dance star of the week" for Kirstie Alley's *100 Days of Dance*. After appearing on *Dancing with the Stars*, Kirstie's goal was to get as many people as possible dancing for a hundred days straight. This dovetailed with Aaron's personal practice of picking up his hoop at least once a day. He made a video and posted it on Kirstie's site. He felt that his style of dance would stand out from the other participants; and he was right. They loved the uniqueness of hoopdance. His video was posted on the home page of the contest website, and the sponsor, Capezio, sent him a gift package that included a pair of dance shoes.

Finally, Aaron was nominee for Youth Hooper of the Year. His parents were taking an interest. "My mom and dad helped me set up a part-time performance career within our local community, and I became an insured stage and fire artist, working on getting my name out there as much as possible." He posted tutorials on his YouTube channel and left his shirt off while teaching shoulder hooping so we could see the way his muscles and bones move.[7] [V]

* * *

After waist hooping, shoulder and knee hooping are core advanced basics. You can begin with tutorials online and practice the tips for shoulders and knees that follow. Then discover variations all your own through personal practice, in classes, and at jams. Nothing takes the place of hooping with people who love it as much as you do.

Hoopdancing teaches us to be fully engaged in our own process, while being equally aware of all that is going on around us. Take advantage of this tool whenever you can, by hooping in unfamiliar territory or public places, and with groups of other hoopers.

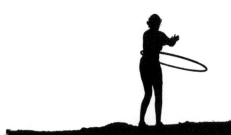

Shoulder Hooping

First learn to raise the hoop from your waist to your chest by moving your rib cage and shoulders more than your hips. Feel the hoop rising to the place where the body is moving most, and use the underarm muscles that we mostly forget we have. Two things will help you get started: a large but not too heavy hoop, and turning in the direction the hoop is moving (to slow down its relative speed so you have more time to react). Bare shoulders and padding on the hoop also help. I cover some of my hoops with cork bicycle-handlebar tape.

- Start by hooping around the waist, moving side to side, then begin to move your rib cage more than your hips and waist, with the energy still coming up from your legs and feet.

- Focus on "chi rising"—feeling your breath energize your chest, keeping shoulders relaxed (not riding up to your ears)—and the hoop will creep up, maybe just an inch or two at first, but keep practicing this.

- Once you can get the hoop up to your chest, use the muscles under your arms to propel it. Accomplish this in both directions before you move on to shoulder hooping.

- With the hoop circling your chest, you can dip your arms into the free space, and the hoop will be on your shoulders.

- With the hoop on your shoulders, use a side-to-side push with a front-to-back roll. Arms are active with elbows fairly close to your sides. Your lower half is moving only to keep the side-to-side pulse, to turn in the direction of the hoop, and eventually to dance.

Review Anah's tutorial from chapter 1, link 4; Aaron's above, link 7; and Caroleeena's in chapter 9, link 1. Caroleeena reminds us to dress for success by leaving shoulders bare.

Above and Below the Knee

Using a spacious and lightly padded hoop, learn to move the hoop gradually down to just above your knees. There are many ways to knee hoop, but I used SaFire's method to start.[8]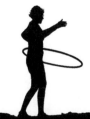

- Begin by hooping around the waist, moving from side to side with your knees fairly close together, and slow down, pulsing with your thighs to bring the hoop just below your derrière. Clear the fleshy part of your buttocks and see if you can keep the hoop there. Turning always helps.

- Once you can hoop on your thighs in both directions, you can bring the hoop lower, keeping knees close together, one slightly bent. Don't spin the hoop on your kneecaps; keep it well above.

- The "standing leg" will carry your weight and the slightly bent "pushing leg" will propel the hoop. If the hoop is traveling from left to right, the left leg stands, and the right leg pushes; from right to left the right leg stands, and the left pushes.

- For me the standing leg is not idle: it pushes in the back with a tiny tap, and the pushing leg pushes in the front.

To take it down another notch, try a kick start: from a standstill with your hoop on the ground, pick it up with the toe of your foot and spring into action. I'm learning this one from a video by Sharna Rose.[9]

Chapter Five Links

www.HoopDanceBook.com/chapter5

1. "Nineteen" by Paul Hardcastle, vinyl. 1985.

2. *Michele Clark on Her Rooftop.* No date.

3. *Hoopdance Book: Renee.* Aug. 10, 2012.

4. *Nadia Sophia—Fire and Hoops—Demo.* Nov. 3, 2009.

5. *Hoop Dance Tutorial: Sustained Spinning Shoulder Duck In.* Oct. 30, 2009.

6. *E.T. Hoop Dance.* Jan. 2, 2012.

7. *Shoulder Hooping Tutorial.* Feb. 4, 2012.

8. *SaFire Hoop Dancing Tutorial: Beginner Knee Hooping.* Jan. 17, 2008.

9. *Kick Start.* Jan. 18, 2007.

SIX

Hoopdance Pioneers

*I arise in the morning torn between a desire to improve
the world, and a desire to enjoy the world.*
—E. B. White, author of *Charlotte's Web*

One band's initiative sparked the imaginations of key individuals from California and New York, Chicago and the little town of Carrboro in North Carolina, Australia and South Africa. Enthusiasts experimented and improvised. Learning as much from their own firsthand experiences as from each other, they stepped outside of what they knew to blaze a trail. Trading in my rocking chair for a pair of dance shoes, I set out to meet them.

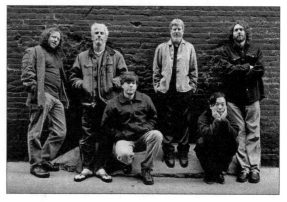

String Cheese Incident ignited the hoopdance movement by introducing their fans to large dance hoops. The band started out in 1993, playing little clubs in Telluride and Preston Butte, Colorado. A few years later, they brought irrigation-tubing hoops decorated with colorful tape to the Telluride Bluegrass Festival. It was a simple gimmick to get people moving, and it worked. The hoop became the band's emblem, and their contracts began to stipulate that hoops be allowed inside the venues they played.

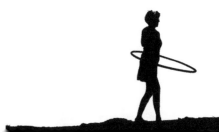

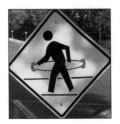

To signal the band's presence in their town, devoted fans altered pedestrian crossing signs, adding a hoop to the figure in the walkway. When the band once played in San Francisco, a hoop-adapted sign marked the crosswalk in front of City Hall, and it stayed there for months after String Cheese Incident had gone. By the early 2000s, fans were bringing their own hoops to concerts, and band members were hooping onstage.[1] [V]

Stepping through the Vortex

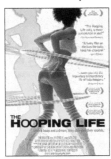

Amy Goldstein is coproducer of the documentary film *The Hooping Life*, which features many of the hoopdancers I interviewed. I had several e-mail exchanges with Amy, but she wouldn't give me her phone number or address until I was in her neighborhood. I didn't take the uncertainty as a negative; meeting the LA contingent of hooping was important, so I was persistent. When I finally arrived at Amy's studio, I got briefed on the film and introduced to Sass Schultz, who was visiting Amy from South Africa on her way to Burning Man (Sass's story of healing from childhood trauma is in chapter 4).

Sass started hoopdancing in her late thirties, when a friend invited her to a Moon Tribe gathering, where people get together in the Southern California desert to play music and dance under the full moon. It

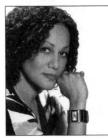

was December 2000. She says, "That's where I saw a tall, skinny woman dancing in the dust with a hoop. I thought, 'Oh, I've got to try that.' My hoop fell to the ground each time I tried, but I couldn't walk away." The beautiful woman showed Sass again and again how to hoop until she got it. Five hours later Sass was still hooping. The woman was Anah Reichenbach, the famous Hoopalicious, and Sass bought two hoops from her that day.

Married and doing her version of "the Hollywood wife of an actor," Sass didn't have to work. But she struggled to find acting jobs because she is, after all, an actor herself. She had been dancing and acting since she was fourteen, two talents that led naturally to performing as a hoopdancer. "Even though I was acting in South Africa, it's very different when you get to Hollywood. Finding the hoop just spun me off in a different direction.

It was fairly addictive, and I had scant competition for fire-hooping performance in Los Angeles at that time."[2] [V]

It was two years before Sass learned to hoop with her upper body,
whereas many coming into the movement now develop entire lexicons
of moves in a matter of months. "For a long time," she says, "larger and
heavier hoops were considered better. When hoopers started playing with
smaller, faster hoops, they began doing things we couldn't have imagined
when we started out." In less than a decade, the insular speciality of hoopdance would dovetail into a whole new world of movement, repurposing
ideas and technique from circus, vaudeville, gymnastics, and sacred ritual.

In 2003 Sass joined the Good Vibe Hoop Tribe with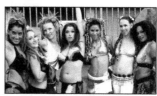
Hoopalicious. The tribe performed for parties such
as Sting's birthday and another organized by Robert
Downey Jr. for his girlfriend, and for Cirque du Soleil's
opening night after-parties.[3] [V]

Performing was only part of the allure for Sass. She is most attracted to
hooping as a leveler of social status: a barista from a coffee shop and a top-
class surgeon are equally qualified for hoopdance. Success is "not about
what you drive or what you wear. It is the rapport you build with the people
around you and how you can rock that hoop. As a synthesis creation, there
is sympathetic likeness amongst hoopers, without sameness."

Before she met Anah Hoopalicious at the Moon Tribe gathering, Sass
had never seen hoops in the Los Angeles party scene. Yet from that day
onward there was hooping at every party she went to. "If you hooped in
Los Angeles at that time, you knew everybody else who hooped. It was a
small circle. You were either taught by Anah or by someone who learned
from her. I call Anah the 'Eve of Hoopers' because she birthed us all."

Anah Reichenbach (Hoopalicious)

Hoopalicious introduced hooping's resurgence to the Los Angeles rave
and club scene, and like a new-wave Johnny Appleseed, she spread the
movement by traveling with her handmade hoops and teaching people
how to use them. She hadn't tried hooping as a child, but when she finally

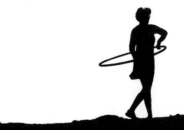

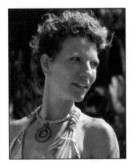

discovered it at a High Sierra music festival in 1997, she found new purpose in her life. Little did she know then the profound effect she would have on so many other people. "It just put me back in child space. Normally I share well, but even though it wasn't my hoop, I was so connected with it I couldn't stop." When people asked her, "Can I use the hoop now?" she said, "No, I'm still using it." But she couldn't take it home.

There were no neighborhood hoop groups, and Anah found no instructions for making hoops. She bought whatever she could find at toy stores, but she couldn't re-create the feeling she was looking for. She called the String Cheese Incident headquarters. She didn't get a knowledgeable person on the phone. It was suggested that she tape together a length of heater hose. That didn't work at all—it was floppy, and the tape wouldn't hold. Then she tried all the tubing and types of connectors (including nails and screws) she could find at hardware stores. When she finally worked out a design that she could hoopdance with, she and her boyfriend, Collin, sold everything they owned, moved into a van, and began to sell hoops on the summer music festival circuit.

The year Sass met Hoopalicious was a high point for Anah and Collin. They sold all their hoops, including the one Anah used. The take of about $4,500 was good money, but it left Anah hoopless on the last day of the trip. As she began to regret selling her personal hoop, she saw the man who bought it standing on a chair, hooping, and holding a sign that read, "Need a ride to Colorado." "He seemed so happy," she says, "I was glad to go without." Her first Hoopalicious demo video is an example of early West Coast hooping style.[4] [V]

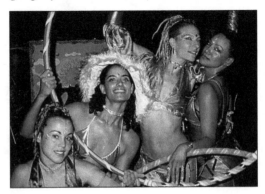

As her practice deepened, Anah discovered what she calls "a cellular connection" with the hoop. "The rhythmic awakening of consciousness that can happen when the hoop communicates with you—body, mind, and spirit—is like nothing else. If you are feeling unsure, the hoop will wobble even when you seem to be physically making all the right moves." State of mind, or some might say the state of your soul, becomes manifest when you hoop. This means that even though you often can't avoid how you feel, when you begin to hoop, you gain the ability to change how you feel, which sometimes you must do in order to hoopdance. If the hoop isn't falling, flying out of your hand, or banging into some part of your body, you may be missing your next revelation. Anah says, "If you want to get to a place of energetic release, you can't hide from what is in your head, and you have to be willing to let the hoop drop in order to find your edge."

When you get stuck in what you do well, try hooping as fast as you can (turning in the direction opposite to that of the hoop) and then very slowly (going with the direction of the hoop) until you find the limits of your ability. Then challenge that edge a little whenever you hoopdance.

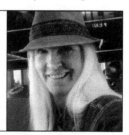

Fran Reichenbach (Anah's Mamalicious) says: "Anah was a shy child and didn't try new things easily. I was surprised when she came home and said she wanted to hoop professionally."

Strength in Numbers

Life, like dancing, is a series of next steps, many of them impromptu. Before there was a hooping industry, only a handful of people thought about hooping as a way of life. Burning Man in 2002 was a turning point, with hoopers reaching a critical mass after which many more people began making and selling hoops, and the demand for dance hoops and teaching grew. Individuals became companies, and companies began to proliferate. Anah explored many avenues of uncharted territory in order to sustain

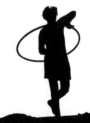

hoopdance as her livelihood. For several years she performed in sexy boo-tie shorts and played to big audiences. She taught classes and eventually established a teacher-training program, in which she helps new teachers connect with students intuitively by sharing both technical and personal introspection skills. She teaches a method of observation that supports the ability to anticipate and solve problems, stressing two points:

- Identify the problems that students may be unable or unwilling to express.

- Be supportive of individuals when addressing problems within a group.

In her work as a mentor Anah encourages hoopdancers to experience the beauty of internal motivation. "As I grow older," she says, "I prefer to hoop my heart out for a few people who happen to be in the right place at the right time." She continually works to bring hooping back to its roots in dancing. To that end she teaches muscle strengthening exercises to facili-tate the fitness conditioning that enables us to dance more freely. Her ath-letic, aesthetic, and personal motivation principles are aimed at developing the maximum potential each of us is capable of with the hoop. I can keep my core strong by doing squats and lunges while hooping, and add stabil-ity by practicing Anah's "ballet steps," even though my own strength and flexibility will never be like hers.[5] V

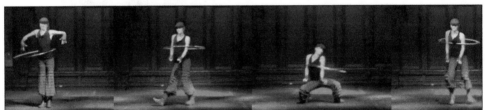

Ballet Steps

Taking a bigger step is an exercise in balance: keeping the chest elevated, navel toward the spine, and pelvis in neutral (sit bones pointing toward the floor, rather than back or tucked forward), with hips and rib cage facing front, even when the legs are in motion. Done as individual steps I regain my balance in between and have time to think about where I am contact-ing the hoop. As I gain balance and strength, this movement becomes more fluid, one step after another, abdominal muscles rolling with the changing contact points. Eventually I may be able to lift each leg in turn, swing my pointed toes high to the side, and sail a leg from back to front without losing my balance, while keeping the hoop on a flat horizontal plane. Not a small thing to strive for.

The ideal is to lift the leg high in back of you, and swing it around to the side and then to the front before putting your foot down. That is one "ballet" step. Practice by making it three steps so you can sense the changes in how your body is contacting the hoop. Start by waist hooping with shoulders aligned over hips, right foot a normal step ahead.

1. Lift your left foot behind you as high as you can. With your weight on the standing leg you are now pushing front to back.

2. Swing the lifted leg out to the side as far as you can, while maintaining your posture of hips and rib cage facing front, which requires a shift to side-to-side contact.

3. As you bring the leg high in front (pushing front-to-back again), step down to complete the step, shifting your weight to the right leg for the next three-part step with the other foot.

Anah's Mamalicious

Anah grew up in Los Angeles. Her father is jazz musician Bill Reichenbach, and her mother, Fran Reichenbach, is a social activist. Fran and Anah, like Ariana and Laura at Hooping Harmony, are family. Being in their presence is like being with childhood friends: they have fun together and support each other. When I met them, Fran came with Anah to 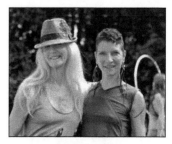 every event where her daughter was teaching. Besides hooping together, they have adorned hats with feathers, made bustle skirts and hooping pants, and dreamed of starting a movement center.

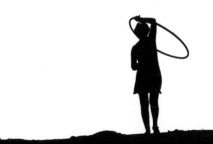

When Fran first tried Anah's hoop, she was barely able to keep it going. With persistence hoopdance helped her get into better shape. Starting with a large hoop, she burned calories fast. As she progressed, she made her hoops smaller and lighter. They were gentler and more suited to her naturally slim physique, and best of all they kept her engaged in learning. "Making your hoop smaller an inch at a time is a good way to challenge yourself. Even a half-inch can make a difference in the way a hoop feels and the amount of energy you expend."

Fran's hoop became more than an exercise tool the first time she viscerally felt a synchronicity between her hips, the hoop, and the music. It was thrilling, and she wanted to share the experience, but she took time to let her changes become integrated in body and soul before hooping in public. "Eventually, the hoop helps you learn balance, poise, and grace—things you don't know you are missing until you start seeing them in yourself."[6] Ⓥ

Rayna McInturf (Hoopnotica)

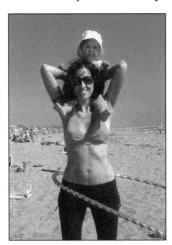

Author of the original Hoopnotica *Preg-O* booklet mentioned in chapter 4, Rayna McInturf first saw hoopdance in 2000. Hoopalicious was dancing on the street at an art festival in the Silver Lake neighborhood of Los Angeles. "I was enthralled," Rayna says, "and I knew right away that I would do it. I bought a hoop from Anah, began to experiment, and we became friends." Rayna thought she was just having fun hanging out with a woman she looked up to as a goddess, but hooping was quietly changing her life. She got really good really fast, and soon she was on stage. "Anah had to drag me into performance. I chose the stage name Hoopnotica, even though I was very hesitant at first. We performed together for several years."

In May 2003 Rayna left the Los Angeles hoopdance community and her full-time job in computer tech support. She went off to New York to discover her own version of the creative life with her boyfriend, Sammy Bliss. She was isolated from other hoopers during the summer and into fall. "Alone I was able to discover and develop my own style of hoopdance and fire-dance performance." She taught classes and waited tables to supplement her income. Then she and Sammy traveled through Europe, visiting five countries in five weeks. Rejoining their Los Angeles community at the end of the year, Rayna reconnected with the growing hoopdance movement as a full-time teacher and performer.

In 2006 Gabriella Redding, who had been a student in Rayna's Hollywood class, joined her in business and became the CEO of Hoopnotica. Their company became one of the largest distributors of fitness hoops in the world. Then during Rayna's pregnancy, she wrote the *Preg-O* booklet. A few months after her daughter, Anjali's, birth, in November 2009, she left Hoopnotica and moved to Northern California with Sammy and Anjali, to focus on her family.

Two years later Rayna and Anah once again joined forces, as partners in Hoop Revolution. Lucky for me they based their company in the San Francisco Bay Area for a time and continued to teach classes and hold jams. Rayna says, "Teaching hoopdance never gets old, especially when the naysayers who believe they can't move their bodies in this way finally get it. They light up. They're like kids again with giant grins on their faces, yelling 'I did it!' and laughing." Now, it's not just Anah and Fran, but Rayna and Anjali as well, coming to events as an extended family unit.

Groovehoops

On the other side of the country in New York City, people learned about hoopdanced from Jesse Kile, one of the Earthlight Players in Ang Lee's 2009 feature film *Taking Woodstock*. She was also the originator of the group that eventually split into Action Hoops and Groovehoops. Loren Binder continued Action Hoops as a fitness program, and Stefan Pildes became most widely associated with the collective Groovehoops, which Jesse describes as a glam-rock hoop circus. "Groovehoops spent five outrageous years touring the U.S. with rock bands like the String Cheese Incident, Sound Tribe Sector Nine, the Brazilian Girls, and George Clinton

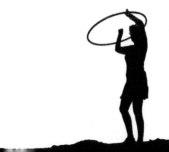

and Parliament Funkadelic." The group is noted for its highly choreographed synchronized hooping.[7]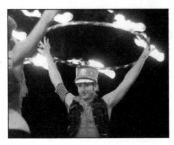

An Ordinary Superstar

At Stefan Pildes's weekly Groovehoops class at the 14th Street Y in the city, Nico had his first real encounter with hoopdance. We practiced with students of all ages. Afterward, Stefan told me about the founding of Groovehoops. "It's a sweet New York story. The day after 9/11, a dozen or so friends gathered together in Central Park, trying to come to terms with what had just happened." They brought things to play with, including hoops. It wasn't the first time Stefan had picked up a hoop, but that day he "gelled" with it and spent hours hooping. A few of the friends returned to the park to hoop the next week. They went again and again, and the group grew from five to fifty within a year. When passersby asked if they were a hula-hooping club, someone said, "I guess so." When asked to sell a hoop, they decided they could make them.

"Can you come teach at my gym?"

"Sure."

"Can you perform at my party?"

"I guess so, yeah."

Stefan and his friends had other skills as well: one was a choreographer, another a stylist, and another a stage manager. Together they casually figured out how to do the things people wanted. Stefan kept tabs on the schedule for rehearsals and performances, and made sure everyone got paid. He became the hoop organizer for New York. If somebody wanted to hire a hooper, they called Stefan. Originally Groovehoops performed theatrical dance shows that he is still proud of. "Jesse Kile, our rehearsal director, was a driven dance major and introduced me to a part of the art world I previously knew nothing about. I was the business guy with a little acting ability, and because of my editing skills I could put together videos that showed our talent."

Stefan had a natural talent for coordinating entertainment. When Rich Porter and object manipulator Rainbow Michael were practicing new hoop patterns in a jam at Hoop Convergence, people started to congregate around them. Stefan jumped in to organize the crowd, transforming Rich and Rainbow's practice session into a performance.

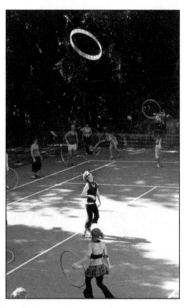

I was at one of Stefan's classes when he came to California. At Hoopcamp he had everyone tossing hoops into the air or across the court to a partner. I'd made it a policy up to that time not to partake in sports where anything comes flying at me, but I played and watched as he demonstrated seemingly impossible throws and catches.

Hooping does not make everyone a celebrity, but in Stefan's little corner of the universe people knew about him. Even in Berlin. He went there because he had heard it was a wonderful, artistic city. Then one night he and his girlfriend had dinner at a friend's favorite restaurant. On their way out, they saw an advertisement of a bear with a hoop around its waist. With their limited German they figured out that there was hooping at a particular club every Tuesday. It was Tuesday, and the club was just three blocks away.

When Stefan arrived, two girls were hooping on the dance floor, and no one else was dancing. "I waited until one of them dropped the hoop and walked on over to pick it up. At first you could see they were expecting the usual drunken guy trying to hoop." But when he started hoopdancing, they exclaimed in unison, "You're Stefan from Groovehoops!"

"How could you know that?" he asked.

"We watch your videos all the time."

The Berlin group of six hoopers, which was about as many as could fit in the bar, was honored to meet Stefan. "That was a great night of hooping in the middle of Europe in the middle of winter that I never could have predicted." His early *How to Groovehoop* video had an international influence.[8] V

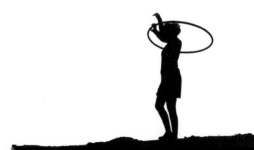

Structured Abandon

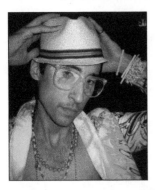

Malcolm Stuart is another original member of Groovehoops. He integrates his love of painting with performance by airbrushing painted "outfits" for himself and others on fabric or directly on the body. By performing in galleries, he recontextualizes hoopdance as fine art without ever losing sight of its true worth. "Hooping has a built-in whimsy," he says. "No matter how seriously I take it, hoopdance remains light and playful. Even when I'm rehearsing or teaching choreography, it is still play."

Despite a slight cold, with clouds and the cityscape as a backdrop, Malcolm hooped for Nico and me on the blustery roof of his building. He performed with amazing agility even though gusts of wind fought him for control of his hoops at every turn. Back in his studio, surrounded by paintings, props, and costumes of all kinds, he told me his life story.

He was a late bloomer. A shy, athletic kid, he developed his spatial awareness and strong body-mind connection playing soccer and basketball in school. Some people saw him as an outgoing youth, but he didn't feel that way. "I remember being at a wedding: older friends dragged me out onto the dance floor, and I thought I was just going to die. I was the classic awkward preteen and couldn't stand people watching me."

All that began to change at age fourteen, when Malcolm got interested in his dad's collection of funk music and started dancing in the privacy of his bedroom. "I can't tell you exactly when I switched to being the one who was breaking the ice on the dance floor. It became a comfortable thing for me to do: to shoulder the scrutiny, with everyone else afraid to be the first one dancing." Later he would use this experience when he was hired to entertain; he would show up at events looking great and festive, and dance as if nobody were watching, even though they were.

At eighteen Malcolm was living at a commune called Universally One in Santa Rosa, north of San Francisco. It was a healing center where members practiced Reiki and yoga, offered nutritional consultation, and threw parties. "That place helped me heal some of the damage of growing up human in an often inhumane culture." Through Universally One he became part of Existdance, a collective of people who loved to move and were inspired by the potential of working together. "We developed shows, providing a framework for each other to grow as people and as performers. That's where I started performing dance, but it took going to New York for me to find hooping."

After spending almost four years at the Santa Rosa Junior College, where he took every course in the art department, he decided to move on. His girlfriend at the time talked about going to New York, which prompted Malcolm to move there and to enroll in the School of Visual Arts. His girlfriend decided to stay in Los Angeles; he looked for a community similar to Existdance, and found it with Groovehoops. The quick, fluid, and quirky hooping style he developed is evidence of his history with teen funk, Existdance, and Groovehoops: with "structured abandon," he throws caution out the door and enters a richly textured unknown.[9]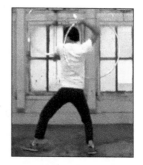

Malcolm first picked up a hoop to dance with at a party in Dumbo (Down Under the Manhattan Bridge Overpass). Jesse Kile was watching. She invited him into her group then and there. "Jesse sat me down on her lap" he admits, "and told me we were going to be friends, and I was going to hoop with her in the park. Then she made me one of the group's 'best friends,' and I moved into their loft."

When differences arose about rules, how pay would be divided, and who could perform with whom, the group split. Malcolm stayed with the Groovehoops contingent. "We had a super-chill groovy style, very slow and inspired by the jam band scene at that time. It was our East Coast moment—different from the rave, house music, and electronic scene that was happening out west, where Anah and her friends were getting hard core with the beats."

Groovehoops played a central role in the growth of hoopdance in New York. No one else was doing shows and classes like theirs. They spread creative hooping wherever they were: on stage, teaching at the Y, as a group in the park, and as individuals. "It was going to happen anyway," Malcolm

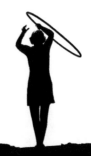

says, "but we were there teaching people, and those people taught people, and so forth. After four years, almost anyone I met hooping around New York I could trace back to Groovehoops."

Later hoopdance began to spread through the Internet, and the greater number of hoopdance events in 2009 made that year another tipping point. Julia Hartsell's second Hoop Convergence in North Carolina brought greater numbers of people together with a wider variety of styles and skills. Staying together in one cabin with other teachers intensified everyone's experience. "Download" was the buzzword they used to describe the learning that was taking place by osmosis. Malcolm says, "I learned something from everyone at that Convergence, in varying degrees and ways. Rainbow Michael's mini hoops expanded my movement vocabulary. Convergence was a doorway to a whole new way of moving."

By the time Malcolm performed for Nico and me on his rooftop, his hoops were as small as they could be and still fit around him. They had challenged his skills with dramatic payoff. For him the porridge is just right when he can work the same hoop around and off his body in perfect smoothness.

Spiraling to the Stars

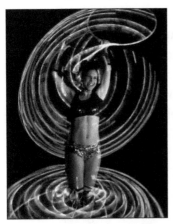

When Vivian Hancock became Spiral, she was catapulted into a life of performance, teaching, and travel. As one of the first hoopdancers to recognize the potential of smaller and lighter hoops, she accelerated the trend to downsize. But the hoop she bought in 2001 at a String Cheese Incident concert was large and heavy: five feet in diameter and made from one-inch tubing.

Spiral twirled her big hoop at many festivals that summer and then brought it back to North Carolina. In Carrboro she became friends with Julia Hartsell and Jonathan Baxter, seeding one of the most receptive places for hooping on the planet. Like Crosby, Stills, and Nash, they influenced each other as much as they individually pushed the boundaries of their craft. Unlike the singers they never performed as a trio.

Julia and Spiral created a fire spinning performance and, after attending a Sufi workshop, they coined the term "sustained spinning." The moves they performed at Hoop Convergence and in online videos, in full, flowing skirts, became a popular style with hoopdancers for years to come. Then Spiral teamed up with Baxter to promote the HoopPath. She says,

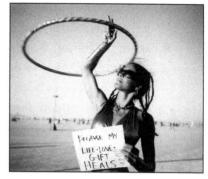

"Baxter and I have taken our work in different directions, but something magical happened between us that opened our creative channels in an exponentially powerful way."

Though Carrboro was Spiral's home base at the time, she visited other hoopers around the country to learn what they were doing. For instance, Anah Reichenbach introduced her to fun fur, the joys of a serger sewing machine, and angle hooping. Spiral says, "I have had the blessing of seeing many hoop styles and had the opportunity to trade tricks." Later, she cocreated Hoop Technique with Rich Porter.

In high school the creative physical outlet available to Spiral had been cheerleading, which created a solid foundation for her later exploration of dance, yoga, climbing, and circus arts. After earning a degree in journalism, she decided that performing was the best use of her talent and passion. She integrates traditional acrobatic and circus techniques with a nontraditional hooping style. "On stage," she confides, "my self-taught self-expression emanates from within and draws on divine connection." Her performance has athletic grace, spiritual awareness, and playful daring. As a first-generation "elder" she is a role model in the hoopdance movement. Flow unlocks her bliss.

During her tutelage at the New England Center for Circus Arts in Vermont, Spiral began to use the smaller hoops that others followed her into. Her tumbling with small hoops created a unique visual effect that required more precise movements. "It has taken years of practice to create a smooth

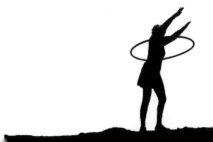

yet dynamic flow with small hoops. The smaller size requires much more turning for hooping on the core." She transformed her hoopdancing from groovy at the 2006 Earth Dance Festival[10] Ⓥ to spinning perfection at the Injuco Gala Show in 2011.[11] Ⓥ

While many performers in the circus and juggling communities work well into their fifties and sixties, Spiral's hooping performance is particularly demanding. As she approached thirty, however, she was not worried about the future. "I'm intelligent and driven, inspired by many things, and I learn quickly. I have no shortage of connections because I make friends easily." A segue to booking agent would be natural. She could also run an entertainment company or teach. "Or," she says, "I could do something completely different—which is more likely."

Hooping Down Under

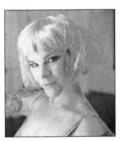

Bunny Hoop Star, creator of the *Hoopy Time Show*, spread hoopdancing in Australia as a "network of consciousness." She says, "Performance is not just about being on stage and receiving applause, it's about sharing a space of happiness. Teaching engages that space as well." Hula hooping is her job in Sydney, where she teaches children after school and adults in the evenings. Otherwise, she spends her time making hoops, performing, and taking bookings for or documenting performances. "It takes a good four years to establish any business," she says, "Mine is a team effort that includes the teachers who work with me and my amazingly talented partner and business mentor, Nick. He designed my logo, and he does much of my marketing."

In Australia hoops were mostly used in the circus, and in the schools for fitness, before three things happened that got Bunny interested in them. In 1995 she saw a performer in a Melbourne nightclub spinning silver hoops all over her body. Next she met a circus trainer in Sydney who taught her some hoop tricks. Later, when she met Anah, Christabel, and Spiral online, hoops became a constant accessory to her new way of life. Bunny and her friends began hoopdancing at parties and nightclubs. "We hooped to the side of the floor where everyone else was dancing without a hoop." At Burning Man, the experience flipped: many people with hoops were dancing together, and there were a few people on the side watching in awe.

At the 2005 Burn, Bunny discovered the style and type of community she wanted to recreate in Australia. "Hoopdance became my Mecca, that hot spot where people spin together in brilliance, moving with courage, intensity, and flow." Dreaming of an inclusive hoopdance community, rather than the exclusivity she perceived in the circus world, Bunny set out to bring people together. Now she has a hoopdance network that reaches from Sydney down to Melbourne and up to Queensland, and is spreading to New Zealand as well. She says, "I have the gorgeous hoop stars in America to thank for that."

Burning Man is an epic trip from Australia, so Bunny decided to create an event in her own desert outback. "I'll bring people into Sydney, then out to the center of Australia, up to Darwin to a festival that happens there, and maybe down to Queensland. It will take time and planning. We'll have a big bus and be super organized." Her group will travel into indigenous communities, staying in each for a few days of creative sharing.[12] [V]

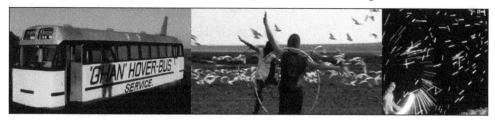

Bunny has been Bunny all her life, with Star attaching itself to her name because of her love of all things astrological. She brought together the Federation of Intergalactic Space Babes (ISB), which she describes as "a collection of hoopy-minded men and women who connect, throughout time in a timeless way inside the hoop, for exploration and a whole lot of bling." They landed at the Sydney Mardi Gras in 2009, eighty strong on the streets of the city, hooping tribal-style in the parade for two and a half kilometers. The ISB attitude? "We're bringing the power back to our individual lives by taking full responsibility for our own happiness, and commanding the level of consciousness that we want to live within."

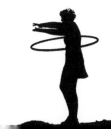

Every class Bunny teaches snaps her energy system into her own space of happiness. Imagine her delight at an opening ceremony of Hoopcamp when she came to California. "With someone as spiritually powerful as Baxter plugging people into their highest state, together amongst the trees, we entered a different world: a space of pure creativity."

The Windy City

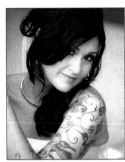

KC Mendicino pioneered hoopdance in Chicago after discovering *poi* in Australia. Starting in Sydney she had little money but plenty of time to hitchhike around and meet people. A man dancing with fire *poi* showed her some basic moves and how to douse the wicks with whiskey to light them on fire. He loaned KC a set of *poi*. "I travelled down to Melbourne and up to Cairns, where he found me again. By then I had learned the fundamentals of fire."

Prior to the early 1960s, fire *poi*
was a private ritual performed by men.

Back in the United States KC's dad made her a set of *poi*. "We cut a soda can and wrapped the aluminum around the end of a dowel and added chain with an eyelet. Dad cut up an old sweatshirt to use for wicks. We had no idea what we were doing, but it worked just fine."

Then KC found a small group of spinners performing in Chicago, who gathered during the full moon to jam on the beach. "I met Elana there. She brought a hoop to the jam, and I thought, 'Okay, this is something I want to do.' Then Elana went off to Burning Man and left her hoop with me." KC taught herself to hoop by watching Anah Reichenbach's first hooping demo. The only video she could find, it inspired her to innovate. She wanted to know, "What is Hoopalicious doing? How could I break it down and take it further?"

KC can manage tricks with two hoops, but she prefers to dance with a single hoop, and fire hooping had the added appeal of being a lot more fire. "I grew up dancing, and fire hoopdance is what I love most." When Elana came back from Burning Man she and KC practiced and performed together as Bellas Fuegas, creating a style of belly dance and fire hooping that was sultry and slow.[13]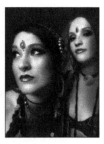

Eventually KC learned of businesses where she could buy ready-made fire gear, but none could top the special fire hoop her dad made. It was a lightweight design that could be decorated to use without fire because its removable wicks screwed out and stored in a travel-safe pouch. "My hoop seemed really small compared to what people were using at Burning Man early on because of the tubing we found, and pretty soon I was selling fire hoops." Those were made from a nine-and-a-half-foot length of half-inch, high-density, maroon-color, 165-psi tubing.

When the best fire dancers were plucked from around the world for the Burning Man Conclave, KC performed with them. Later she performed with Spiral at the NASA Ames Research Center in Moffett Field in California. "Evidently the government didn't think our generation was paying enough attention to space travel, so they threw a big, all-night party to get people interested." It was the first time a rave took place in a government facility. The Chicago-based American electronic band Telefon Tel Aviv was there. They invited KC to perform with them in Israel. Then she met Christabel online. Through a Tribe.net e-mail exchange they arranged to meet at the Winter Music Conference in Miami.

Though many people who meet through the Internet may never converse face to face, KC says, "There is a common denominator of admiration for hooping that goes across state lines and makes us famous to one another. When I introduce myself in person or online, all I have to say is that I hoopdance too." KC never had the sorority-sisters experience, but she is in the hoopdance sorority and can recognize a hoop sister on the street by the clothes she wears and the way she moves. "I want to know her, and I do get to know her, through curiosity rather than competition. In hooping there is an 'everybody up' mentality."

KC was teaching classes regularly in Chicago in 2005, when she helped a young female student recover from a traumatic experience that had left her constantly on guard. After being mugged on the city's South Side by a group of young boys who held her at gunpoint, the student used

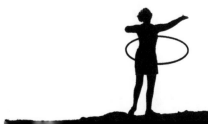

hoopdance to rebuild trust in herself and reclaim her personal boundaries. "You need a little extra space with a hoop," KC says with a gentle flick of her wrist. "Excuse me, could you just move over there a little more?"

KC says: "Bring hooping to schools! It is physical activity, and not everybody wants to kick a ball. Why not give young people a choice that makes them smile?"

When KC met Baxter at Burning Man, he was wearing all white. They hooped close to each other, talking to keep warm. If she had to imagine what hoopdancing should look like for a man, she says, "I couldn't come up with anything better than Baxter's style. He's rough, graceful, and very manly. He is original." As KC was slowing down her own involvement with hoopdance, Baxter and many others were bringing community together outside of Burning Man, not only to learn technique from each other but to share a common meditation on why we gravitate to hoopdancing.

HoopPath Evolution

Jonathan Livingston Baxter (Baxter) is one of the trailblazers profiled in *The Hooping Life*. From his small hometown of Carrboro he travels to teach and preach, but his regular weekly class has rarely been canceled because he doesn't have to be at every class himself. His local followers hold a hoop jam in the classroom space when he's not there. And when he is in town, he says, "If I'm conscious, I'm in class."

When I visited Baxter in Carrboro, I attended his Warrior Class and saw why having a substitute teacher would be difficult. Baxter's words and his delivery of them are as important as his approach is unique. "Through practice we build trust," he says, "not only with the hoop, but with other human beings, creating more genuine relationships. I pass my rhythm on to the hoop, and the hoop passes it back. When the two rhythms are moving together, there is a balance." [14] V

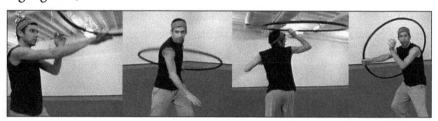

Baxter grew up in Charlotte, but he doesn't think that city could ever become the hooping Mecca that is Carrboro, which he sees as an anomaly within North Carolina. "Carrboro is a hub of liberalism amidst an ocean of conservative thinking. With an 'Old South,' nondance mentality on all sides, our community is compressed and radicalized further." Because people in Carrboro were already used to looking outside the box for new ways of doing things, it was a perfect place for the hooping movement to flourish.

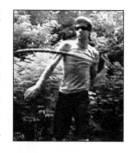

When Baxter first saw Julia Hartsell hoopdance, he had thought of it as "her thing." Then he broke his collarbone. "That's when my own hoop story began, as exercise for an atrophied shoulder." He started using a blindfold because the square of his backyard, where he practiced, was open to the street and passersby interrupted his concentration. In darkness he made a simple and transformative discovery: his body could communicate directly with the hoop.[15] [V]

Then Baxter "buddied up" with Spiral and began a friendly, unspoken competition, hooping to hip-hop music. With it came the bravado of hip-hop dance, which pushed Baxter further into his own "hoopnosis," discovery and understanding acquired through his personal relationship with the hoop. "Spiral and I were each other's biggest fans. It was like being on a sports team with an intrasquad opponent in a competitive field. When it's finally game time you're glad that competitor is by your side."

When Baxter started hooping, he was very opinionated. "I was excited and started talking about 'community' before I could really see one. But once you give a name to something, it helps to shape it." Baxter was the HoopPath teacher. The technique that grew out of his philosophy was demonstrated by Spiral. Baxter says, "Spiral is a woman with broad shoulders. She would wear cute little outfits and then bust out warrior-like moves. She 'mothered' the warrior style. I wrote the HoopPath, but without Spiral it wouldn't have gone anywhere as fast as it did."

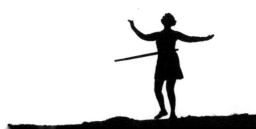

Baxter and Spiral talked about the HoopPath as if it were an established program and Carrboro *the* place for hooping. Their successful promotion started with the attitude that you have to act like you're the best for people to think you're the best. Like a farmer talking about how good his corn is while it is still growing in the field: he looks at the potential of his crop and says, "It's going to be good." From the little town that few hoopers had ever heard of came videos of a style of hoopdancing that seemed radically new.

Meditating on the healing potential of hooping, Baxter invented mythological stories of the Maidan that he found useful to help his students both get in flow and guide their lives. The Maidan, an order of holy women from another dimension, are brought to earth by the sacred circle that connects them with the spirit world in nature. Hooping is their energy source. The rhythm of the hoop brings them back to the tides and flow from which they derive their peaceful yet formidable power.

The Maidan (pronounced "myDAN") is Baxter's fictitious
ancient culture of women and nature,
which is neither religious nor strictly for women.

The Maidan exist within a vast system of complex rhythms, and the hoop is their tool for understanding themselves and what they give to the world. There are practical insights at the heart of Baxter's teaching, such as "relationships create a third rhythm." He says, "I have a rhythm, my partner has a rhythm, and together we create *pe*a*ce* [a Maidan term pronounced "peAHchay"]. The third rhythm takes you both further than you could go on your own."

The Maidan have "sun sides" and "tree sides" as well as first and second currents. These directions help orient students to the movement Baxter teaches. When there is receptivity to his stories, HoopPath classes flow, but not everyone understands metaphor. Of those who do, some embrace the Maidan legend personally. More pragmatic students can get caught up wondering about the details of when all this happened, C.E. or B.C.E.? Others might take it for a cult in which Baxter holds the rulebook. In truth the HoopPath is open source. Each student writes his or her own story within the framework of the Maidan cosmology, and the application of fantasy sometimes becomes a form of personal therapy. In Baxter's own story, a mother, after hearing of her husband's death, screamed so loudly that she deafened herself. The women of the Maidan read the mother's thoughts and transferred them to the character Baxter identifies with, her son.

Baxter and his twin sister were seven months old when their father divorced their mother. At eighteen the twins had a disagreement. They didn't speak to each other for the following sixteen years. During that time each started hoopdancing independently of the other. Then one Christmas they finally had a conversation, and it was about hooping.

Mining Beauty

A born preacher, Baxter uses hoopdancing as a way to indulge in "spreading the word" without having a church or defining a faith. But there are moments when he has doubts. "At first I wondered if I could really teach people how to dance when I was just learning at thirty-five years old! Then someone sent an e-mail that said, 'You don't know me, but I watch your videos, I've read your story, and I've learned to hoop.' That gave me confidence."

Baxter's HoopPath DVD helps students turn their focus toward internal beauty, richness, and wisdom. When he started teaching he thought of beauty as a superficial dressing. Over the years he has come to see it as a radiant feeling rather than an external judgment. "If I *feel* beautiful, I *become* beautiful, and others feel it too." He sees video as a way to reach those who will never come to class. "There are hoopers out there who will only dance in privacy. They don't like to be in public; they will never go to a hoop jam or come to one of my workshops. The Internet has the potential to reach these delicate flowers and maybe even to draw them out of the greenhouse."

In Baxter's program he urges each person to move from the place "wherein his or her truest rhythms lie." There is a woman who comes to his class about once a month, and waist hoops all the way through. "That's what she needs, and that's what she does. She doesn't ask, 'Is this too simple for somebody?' She's her own muse, her own motivation. The

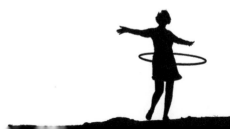

funny thing is, I can tell that others in the class want to be there; they wish they could just waist hoop, but for them it would be boring." The moral is, yield to what you enjoy, write your own meditative practice and physical regimen, and develop your own style. Baxter's is unique and personal, with beautiful footwork that keeps him grounded.[16] [V]

Chapter Six Links

www.HoopDanceBook.com/chapter6

1. *StringCheese2007.mov.* Feb. 18, 2012.

2. *Sass Neck Knee and Ankle Fire Hooping.* May 22, 2006.

3. *The Good Vibe Hoop Tribe.* Jan. 16, 2007.

4. *Hoopalicious Demo!* Jun. 18, 2006.

5. *Bristol Performance.* Jan. 19, 2012.

6. *Mamalicious.* Nov. 11, 2009.

7. *Groovehoops Step To It.* Apr. 11, 2007.

8. *How To Groovehoop.* 2006

9. *Malcolm Stuart Reel 2011.* Jan. 15, 2011.

10. *Spiral @ Earth Dance Festival.* Oct. 1, 2006.

11. *INJUCO 2011 GALA Show Spiral.* Feb. 21, 2011.

12. *Earth Dreaming.* Sep. 2, 2008.

13. *Bellas Fuegas @ Kira's Oasis.* Dec. 29, 2007.

14. *Off-Body Hooping with Baxter from the Hoop Path.* Dec. 25, 2009.

15. *Feelin' it. (Ceelo Green "Living Again.").* Jul. 17, 2006.

16. *Baxter core hoops (mostly) to "Night Falls" by Booka Shade.* Dec. 19, 2009.

SEVEN

Gathering the Tribe

People don't stop playing because they get old;
they get old because they stop playing.
—George Bernard Shaw, playwright

Community is a big part of the attraction of hoopdance. People meet
at a growing number of events. Participants and teachers swap tips and
tricks face-to-face, get inspired, and build collective expertise. Many
hoopdancers travel internationally to hoop with old friends and to make
new ones. Locally hoopdancers meet regularly at jams. And online, single
artists inspire thousands every day through messaging, forum groups, and
video sharing. Every year more hoopdancers meet at Burning Man, the
temporary community based on radical self-expression that is constructed
in the Black Rock Desert of Nevada each fall.

Burning Old Man Gloom

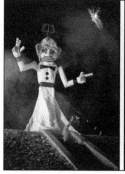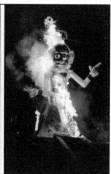

When I lived in Santa Fe, New Mexico,
from 1979 to 1987, I attended the annual
Fiesta, which had been celebrating harvest
season by burning the effigy of Zozobra,
Old Man Gloom, since 1924. In San Francisco, I was surprised to find an artist's
version of this ritual. I went to the fourth
annual Burning Man ceremony, held at
Baker Beach in 1989. The audience had

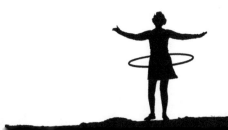

grown from its original collection of friends to three hundred spectators. The Man, built entirely of wood, had grown from his original eight-foot height to an ambitious forty feet that year. The structure buckled prematurely, burning in a semi-erect position. Police looked on with anxiety but didn't stop the burn, and every year it has just kept growing. [1] Ⅴ

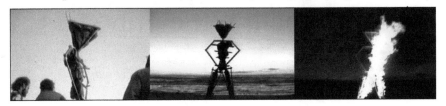

The Playa Burn

In 1991 the Burn moved to the vast empty space of the playa in Nevada, eventually establishing its home in the annual rebuilding of Black Rock City. All evidence of the town's existence is removed after each festival. Its population doubled each year from 1993 to 1996, when it accommodated over eight thousand participants. Many String Cheese Incident fans went to the Burn, so there were hoopers there from the start. But they didn't always find one another because their numbers were small and the festival covered a large area of desert.

When Julia Hartsell (Jewels), founder of Hoop Convergence in North Carolina, went to her first Burn, the forty-foot man stood securely atop a forty-foot geodesic dome, and there were over thirty-five thousand participants. It was August 2004, but even then Julia was disappointed, because initially she didn't see anyone else with a hoop. There was plenty of music, though, so she hooped alone until she met up with Stefan and Malcolm from Groovehoops. Then they found Baxter, Spiral, and other core hoopdancers at Center Camp and created a jam that was videotaped by the Groovehoops crew. [2] Ⅴ

In 2008 the Burning Man temporary town covered
five square miles—nearly the spread of San Francisco.
By 2010 the crowd peaked at 51,525 participants,
with a record number of hoopers in attendance.

Burning Man wasn't the convergence Julia had hoped for. She wanted to learn more than tricks; she wanted to hear about the heartfelt experience of other hoopers. "I was looking for deep connection, something intimate. Burning Man was the wrong venue. It was too big, and its mission was too broad."

Creating Hoopdance Events

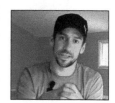

Baxter was already teaching his HoopPath program when he wrote an impassioned Internet plea to the hooping community in the summer of 2007. "It was not long after the Iraq war had gotten ugly. I invited hoopers around the world to become part of a positive rhythm generation. It was a weekend in Carrboro, North Carolina, built by hoopers, for hoopers." Eighteen men and women, including Southern California's Diana Lopez (Body Hoops), who was well known as the creator of the Infinity Hoop, came from afar. Baxter and Spiral, his HoopPath partner at the time, picked guests up at the airport. "We charged a hundred bucks for the whole weekend and housed them in our homes," Baxter recalls. "I was on cloud nine. We also had locals, so there were about twenty-five students in the workshops."

The next year Baxter and Spiral rented a bigger space, expecting to accommodate forty people. They sold thirty-four tickets the day they went on sale. After nine days they began scrambling to find beds for eighty people. The HoopPath's demographic includes many women in their forties and fifties. Baxter wanted it to be a vacation for them as well as a training course. "We put everybody up somewhere—even camping. The next year we reserved a block of rooms at a hotel and had a hundred and forty participants."

Hoop Convergence

In 2008 Julia Hartsell convened the first annual Hoop Convergence in North Carolina's rolling green countryside. Like Baxter's HoopPath retreat, it offered skill sharing, classes, and jams. Unlike the HoopPath, Julia's event hosted a wide range of hoopdancers to share the variety of their expertise and philosophy.

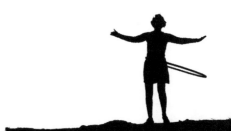

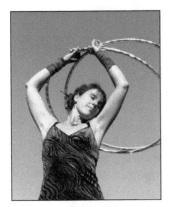

Julia and her partner, drummer Scott Crews (profiled in the music section of chapter 9), founded the
Flojo movement space in Carrboro. They hosted Nico
Gerbi and me during our visit there. Julia had danced
for us in her tiny living room, and we were mesmerized by her twin silver hoops whirling up and down
her body until they locked overhead like a spinning
globe for the finale.

The 2008 Hoop Convergence changed the hooping
landscape and became a model for the many retreats
that followed it. Meals are tasty and healthy. Some classes are straightfor-
ward, while others demand thinking outside the hoop, and a few offer
games to help you master tricks. AcroYoga, *poi,* and other flow arts are
on offer, and the setting sun brings out the LED hoops, fire, and performances. Custom clothing, hoops, and other props are available for pur-
chase, and live music is played throughout the festival until the closing
circle. Convergence brings veteran hoopers together with new students,
opening the conference with a circle of more than one hundred and forty
participants. They camp out or stay in cabins, and the Hoopers' Ball takes
place on a solar-powered stage.

The idea for the first Hoop Convergence began to germinate in a dis-
cussion group online. Julia, Caroleeena, and Spiral, with a few others in
North Carolina and Revolva in Oregon, began to shape the event by talking about what kinds of classes were needed. Greg Roberts, an AcroYoga
teacher and traveling artist from Burning Man, created the logo and built
the initial website. The date was set for a five-day retreat. Julia called Stefan
Pildes of Groovehoops in New York, and he committed to attending. Anah
Reichenbach was in a low period and unsure, but when the time came, she
arrived from Los Angeles.

Anyone who submitted a well-thought-out proposal was invited to
teach. Ariana and Laura Marie were there from Hooping Harmony. Laura
says, "Hoop Convergence was the very first event of its kind. It was poi-
gnant and beautiful to watch so many people with different backgrounds
come together." Shakti Sunfire came from Colorado and prophesied, "We
are going to miss the intimacy of this first gathering." Others came from
the Midwest, Alaska, and Canada, yet the group was small enough that

after the opening circle Julia knew everyone's name. Her own vision for hoopdance is spiritual and holistic, and her event was heartfelt. It was also chaotic because everyone was in every class, and sticking to the schedule became less important than what they were doing. Julia says, "If something really juicy happened, we just kept playing with it."

Hoop Convergence doubled in its second year. Julia learned to use a spreadsheet to keep track of participants, shortened the event to four days so that more people could attend the full program, and received more proposals for classes than she could accommodate. Some of the first-year teachers returned, and some first-year participants became teachers. What the 2009 gathering lost in intimacy it gained in energy. The live music and hoop jams every night amazed even Julia.[3] [V]

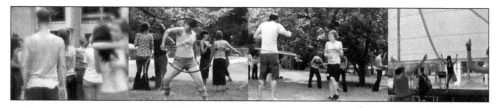

Julia's Story

As a child Julia had taken pottery classes, turning clay on a wheel, and had twirled with joy while dancing. As an adult she was drawn to the circular meditation of hoopdance. Two weeks after 9/11, she saw Spiral for the first time, hoopdancing at a music festival, but was too shy to approach her. The next time they met Julia introduced herself to Spiral, and learned that they lived close to each other in Carrboro. They became instant friends, getting together to sew, have dinner, go to shows, and hoop.

Julia learned to do tricks like lifting the hoop off her waist so she could continue hooping while doing little tasks like lowering the flame under a pot of soup on the stove. When she saw a belly dancer urge a hoop up and down her core without using her hands, she taught herself to do it. She hadn't thought about hoopdance as a profession until she saw a burlesque hooper from the Bindlestiff Family Circus use multiple hoops at a little club in Carrboro. Julia was brought onto the stage to hoop and to throw hoops

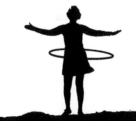

onto Miss Saturn, who made her living by hooping at birthday parties and in burlesque shows, using toy hoops that she decorated with tape. Julia made a hoop big enough for two people to occupy at once for Miss Saturn to use in her act.[4] V

Then Julia and Spiral lived together for a year and a half, hooping hard core. They made costumes and hoops, and taught at the Weaver Street Market, a spot for community gatherings in Carrboro. They held a day camp for kids in a yoga studio and offered a few classes at a fitness center. Eventually they created a fire-hooping act to perform professionally. At their first audition Julia recalls standing in the back of the venue wondering, "How did this happen—that I am about to light something on fire in a dining room! As a kid I hated recitals, but here I am, and it is all happening so fast."

Later, at the Winter Music Conference, a networking event for DJs and musicians, Julia met Anah Reichenbach (Hoopalicious) and Rayna McInturf (Hoopnotica), who had been hired to perform. They showed her the wonderful costumes they had brought, but they didn't get to wear them. Instead they were given bikinis, and their bodies were airbrushed with the logo for Bacardi, one of the conference sponsors. Seeing women she held in high regard treated that way made Julia vow, "It's not the path I'm walking." She left the ongoing fire performance act to Spiral and took time out to meditate on what the hoop meant to her and what she wanted to do with it. She practiced dervish twirling and began to perform in the art-dance community. "The hoop helped me to create a persona that is positive and participatory, and Hoop Convergence eventually became what I had been looking for at Burning Man: a place to form close relationships with a large number of hoopdancers."

International Events in California

As a novice hooper in 2009 I had my first group adventure at a marathon

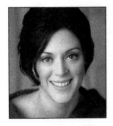

movement-arts weekend put on by Rosie Lila (Miss Rosie). She caught the hooping bug at Burning Man in 2005 and dreamed of being a rock star. Instead, she became a hoopdance performer, teacher, and founder of the Movement Play Microfestival, which she describes as a place to open our hearts and get in touch with our physical selves. Miss Rosie says, "Hooping is a journey for practicing the way we want the world to be, and the way we want to be in it. Letting go of proprietary feelings has been a growth process for me, as I realize that no one owns the hooping movement." Her performance is open source.[5] [V]

The 2009 Movement Play was an interdisciplinary summer campout in Northern California. After setting up my tent, I wandered the grounds. The dry air was filled with birdsong and electronic beats. Throughout the weekend there were ongoing classes in hooping, yoga, spin toys, and even collage, with DJs spinning music well into the night.[6] [V]

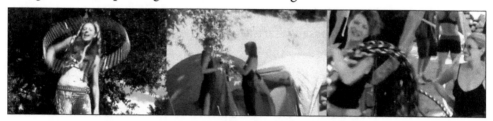

The camp's classroom areas were shaded with colorful triangles of canvas. Resting stations included a geodesic dome, a teepee, and a lean-to with fluffy quilts. The teahouse was a quiet space with a low wooden bar, and anyone could take a clothing-optional dip in the pond or hot tubs at any time. Participants were encouraged to move and relax their bodies, and to take personal responsibility as well. Everyone signed up for a work task, such as helping to cook and serve food. Meals were healthy and delicious because, like many in the hooping movement, Miss Rosie believes in nutritious food that tastes good.

After three short days I had an answer to the most frequently asked question: "What will I get for my $350?" It was an experience that led me, by small steps and choices, to unleash my playful self. On the final evening, while the band Tropo played their mix of live instruments and electronic sounds, I gave in, relinquishing premeditation to play in a velvet mosh of fifty ecstatic dancers. I didn't see the contact improv start but was soon caught up in the gentle pushing and tumbling of one dancer and then the next.

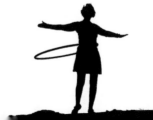

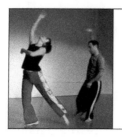

In contact improvisation, two or more moving bodies improvise their combined physical relationships in spontaneous movement. A lovely example is by Kristin Horrigan and Spirit Joseph.[7] Ⓥ

After contact dancing, four artists shared their talent and expertise. Miss Rosie and Hoopalicious gave an incredible hoopdance performance, followed by Tropo's base guitarist, Grant Leonard, in a hooping duet with Isopop's Rich Porter.[8] Ⓥ

As the gathering dispersed I spied an outrageously large geisha whom I suspected to be Ken Masters, then husband to Miss Rosie, sweeping up. Over six feet tall, the hefty figure glided to the teahouse with clandestine grace in black wig, makeup, and kimono. I followed and sat at a low curving table with the four other campers who had been attracted along with me. The mute and somewhat disgruntled geisha prepared tea, served snacks to the guests she liked, and punished the others by throwing them bodily out, albeit gently, into the darkness. Campers were not obliged to take part in this impromptu ritual theater (most didn't know it was happening), but I'm glad I didn't miss it.

Hoopcamp in the Santa Cruz Mountains

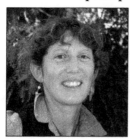

Hoopcamp is the brainchild of Heather Troy, and it takes place in the Santa Cruz Mountains in California. It is a well-organized, fast-paced, four-day weekend offering intensive workshops on a tight schedule to a large number of participants. It bears out my theory that hoopdance culture draws on the best of what the 1960s and 1970s gave us—sharing, caring, and an openness to new experiences with an elevated consciousness. Heather envisions the typical Hoopcamp guest as "a most creative and wonderful individual who seeks out amazing experiences by gathering with like-minded hoop geeks, dancers, and groovy body movers and shakers." It has been one of the largest and most super-charged gatherings of hoopdancers outside of Burning Man.

The year I attended there had been some overbooking (hooping is inclusive), and four had been assigned to my two-person cabin, but soon space was found for everyone. There was a cocktail reception held in the main building where meals were served, and we were shown a few pre-release scenes from the documentary film *The Hooping Life.* After that it was a whirlwind of classes with a break for shopping from vendors, taking a swim, or getting a massage. I bought a custom hoop made by Hoopalicious, and hooping pants by Ahni Radvanyi to go with it. There weren't many people using the pool, so I indulged in one of my hippie cultural traditions: swimming nude before lunch. I found respite there from the cacophony of music, conversation, and laughter.[9] V

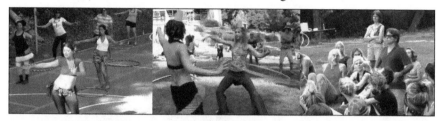

In 2010 Hoopcamp moved to the Pema Osel Ling Tibetan Buddhist Retreat, also located in a redwood forest in the Santa Cruz Mountains. Heather says, "We are blessed to play within the mandala and peace stupa the community has created here, to spin fire in a spiritual place, and to eat meals made from the local bounty of Santa Cruz organic farms." The space has camping, RV hookups, bunk cabins, and two large houses with indoor bathrooms and showers. Rich Porter and Grant Leonard build its temporary structures with lighting and sound. Grant says, "We create environments we like to be in ourselves, and the hoop is always part of the events we support. 2012 is our fifth year at Hoopcamp."

Camp and Jam at Harbin Hot Springs

The Harbin Hoop Jam (also known as Hoop Heaven) is a weeklong event at the Harbin Hot Springs retreat center near Calistoga, California. The event was founded by Patrick Deluz, creator of the LED PsiHoops, so lots of brightly lit late-night play went on there.

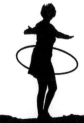

For centuries, before Harbin's unique setting with its miles of hiking trails became a resort in the late 1800s, the indigenous population of the area considered the land and waters to be sacred. Two natural hot springs continue to feed the resort's pools. During the event I had a comfortable 1920s-style room with a shared bathroom in the Harbin Hotel, located across a stream from the conference center where the hoop jam took place. Others camped in areas surrounding the center, or slept on bedding in the carpeted room adjacent to the main hall. The conference center has its own kitchen, used to prepare meals that we unanimously agreed were "shockingly good," and its two private pools were clothing optional.

The polar opposite of Hoopcamp, the jam was a freewheeling, informal respite, and many of the participants were decompressing from hectic schedules. Gail O'Brien, founder of the Manchester Hoop Congress, says, "This camp mirrors the style of U.K. skill sharing more than any other California event. There are no structured classes to separate students from teachers. Everyone learns by playing together." [10] [V]

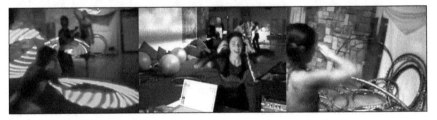

The first Harbin Hoop Jam had sixteen participants. There were twenty-four the second year. I attended the third year with a group of forty, which seemed to be the perfect number. The main hall is large and cathedral-like, so we had plenty of space to play. The wood floor was ideal for dancing, and carpeted sections were great for yoga, tumbling, and martial arts.

Nayeli Michelle Bouvier was our guide to playful exercise and information about bodywork techniques, but group activities left ample free time over the five-day period for friends to develop moves, such as a new way to weave twin hoops. Jo Mondy came from Australia. She moderates the instructors' forum on Hooping.org and showed us how to use twin hoops like a helicopter. [11] [V]

At Harbin I learned to play volleyhoop with no net, which required batting a beach ball with the edge of my hoop. I also tried exercise-ball surfing, in which you line up three or more balls (big enough to be used as chairs) and then fling yourself onto them to glide recklessly across the room. Patrick hooped while standing on one of these balls. Three together became a pseudo roller cart, for playing dodge 'em. Then Tammy Firefly put up her aerial lyra and fabric for everyone to use.

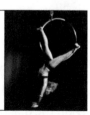

Lyra is a steel ring suspended from a ceiling and used by artists to perform acrobatics

Zach Fischer (Number Nine in the Vegetable Circus) hooped upside-down while hanging from the ring by his knees. Marria Grace of the Boston Hoop Troop (Madame Spinach in the Vegetable Circus) gave a comical performance using a hoop and a parasol. Paired as twins, her empty hoop was filled in many ways while her parasol provided a surface that contracted and expanded with an up, a down, and a handle.

Throughout the week, learning specialist Heather Toles dazzled us with glittering flowers painted on her pregnant abdomen, Adelaide Marcus and Sam Salwei blended aspects of belly dancing, hooping, and partner yoga, and there was exotic chocolate to share. Tiana Zoumer (Wanton) astonished us with her mime and hooping isolations.[12] [V]

Melanie Pleasure was an inspiration. She had liberated herself from a family history of obesity, diabetes, and hypertension by chang-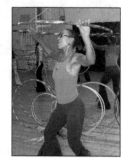ing her focus from acting and accounting to fitness. First she became a gym instructor to help others with the process of becoming physically fit. Then she saw hoopdancing at a fitness convention. It changed her concept of the term "workout." She decided, then and there, "That's for me." She went on to teach hoopdance classes in Southern California. At the end of the 2011 jam, Patrick passed Melanie the jam's organizing baton, and the event was renamed Harbin Flowjam.

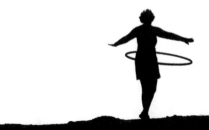

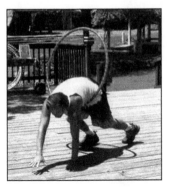

Throughout the year, Van (pronounced "Von") Maffei offered a weekly hoop jam at Harbin Hot Springs. He lived about four miles from the nearest small town. "Isolated from other hoopers, it's easy to feel like I'm king. When the hooping world comes to Harbin, it's humbling. It opens me up to things that are not natural for me, like off-body hooping moves."

He taught us a move he calls the Harbin Hustle, using the downward-dog yoga pose. Keeping his feet planted firmly while waist hooping, he leans forward with the hoop spinning on the diagonal plane. His arms are out in front; then he drops down to place his palms on the floor, bottom in the air, still pumping the torso. The hoop keeps on circling. For an added kick, without missing a beat, he lifts one arm into the air, turning his body sideways, and continues pumping to keep the hoop going. Pretty spectacular.

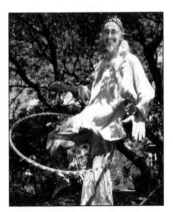

The jam's mentor, Patrick Deluz, is sometimes called Merlin because of the visual magic he brings to hoopdance. Born in Brazil, he lived most of his early life in a private rural paradise. He grew up with no electricity, which meant no TV, radio, refrigerator, or batteries. His toys were a ball and a stick. His company was nature. He describes it as "perfection!" He encountered hula hooping when he came to California and was already in his fifties. "I had always been in love with play, dance, and movement, and when someone showed up at a local dance jam with a large hoop, I was entranced. It was a slice of a ball you could step into—another contact dance partner. Wow!"

In a typical week Patrick might go to a Tuesday night hoop class and hoop on Saturday at the park. On Sundays he attends Dance Church, a spiritual dance jam he helped establish, at which the DJ is the minister, music is the sermon, and dancers are the congregation. But the bulk of his time is spent making and developing hoops. "I probably spend six hours a day, seven days a week, making hoops. Sometimes it's tough, but mostly it doesn't feel like work." It's his meditation, service, passion, and hobby all rolled into one. (See PsiHoops in chapter 9.)

In his martial arts practice Patrick uses swords, but he prefers the hoop for its shape. "It mirrors other circles that appear to us daily—in each other's eyes and in the sun and the moon. A hoop is a kind of minimalist ball, or a sword curled into itself like the Ouroboros, the ancient symbol of regeneration. Swords make good movement partners, but bringing a sword to a dance jam might be seen as threatening." At the dance he rolls hoops onto the floor or throws them to others. Playfully catching their attention, he invites dancers who may be isolated in their own routines to interact with each other and the musicians.

Community Jams

Jams are generally informal meetings where two or more hoopdancers come together to inspire each other. This type of gathering provides individuals with a way to work on personal technique, at their own pace, in the presence of supportive company. Jams foster improvisation and collective growth by offering us an opportunity to let go of the rational thought we use in structured classes, to play, and to make discoveries.

The jam's atmosphere of freedom comes in many forms. Carrboro, North Carolina, offers two types. The Weaver Street Jam congregates informally on the green lawn of the community park, where live music is provided for the entire town to enjoy. The season lasts four or five months each year as weather permits. The more focused HoopPath Jam is held in a rented studio. The indoor space allows hooping year-round, regardless of the weather. This jam got started when HoopPath teacher Ann Humphreys began posting videos of her regular practice. Her peers were inspired to make a weekly jam their priority because they could see that her consistent improvement came from allotting enough time to practice.[13] V

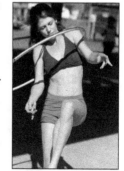

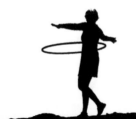

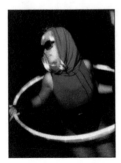

In Berkeley, California, Nicole Wong started the Cherry Hoops' Monday night hoop jam. "After I began teaching hoopdance, I realized that although I was spending a good deal of time inside my hoop, it had been a while since I hooped purely for myself, and I missed that." The jam she established brought together about twenty hoopers of various experience levels in a large aerial dance studio at the Sawtooth Building. Besides the core of regulars, each week brought newcomers who found out about it by word of mouth. Hoop Revolution took up the jam for a while, moving it to the Seventh Heaven Yoga studio, when Nicole moved to San Francisco and joined the Bay Area Hoopers (BAH) at their weekly jam. BAH has been meeting in San Francisco parks in good weather, and indoors in winter, since 2003.[14] [V]

In Memphis, Hooper Troopers jam, give demonstrations, and sell hoops at their local farmers' market. They inspire boys and girls to exercise. Megan Simpson says, "It isn't much good to tell a five-year-old that exercise is healthy for his or her heart, but you can say, 'Hey, let's play with this hoop!'" Her ultimate goal is to open a studio called One More Spin, which is what the kids always say when it's time to stop hooping.

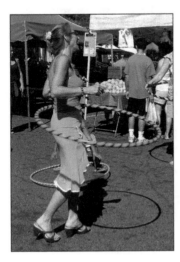

At farmers' markets like the one Betty Lucas frequents in Alameda, California, people are interested in living healthfully.

Jon Coyne (Hoopsmiles) attended the weekly spin jam in Seattle, when he started hooping in 2009. "Soon after my first experience, I met a woman from Cannon Beach, Oregon, who goes by the name Aunt Jess. She taught me my first real hooping tricks." Jon teaches many of those tricks on the Internet. He says, "What I really enjoy about hooping is that it doesn't matter if I'm mad or sad; however I choose to be, I can turn on some music and discover myself in hooping." His "How to Hoop" rap song single is in the iTunes store, and on the video he hoops with Sponyang.[15] V

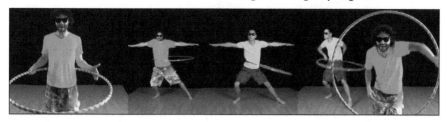

Worldwide Hooping

Becky Lawrence was introduced to hooping by her brother; now their whole family hoops. "My mom, aunt, and I are avid hoopdancers. My aunt teaches hoopdance on Mercer Island in Washington; my mom and brother live in Minnesota. We all stay in touch through the Internet." It is an intergenerational, friends-and-family affair that connects people locally and strengthens long-distance bonds.

The Internet

Hoopdancers share videos online and take part in forum discussions (where individuals start or join a thread by posting messages and replies) and in live chats (real-time discussions with messages that are instantly visible). It is social networking, on the ground and growing. When Tribe.net appeared in 2003, its primary focus was the San Francisco Bay Area, but the Hoop Tribe attracted members from all over the world. It was integral to developing hoopdance. The people who shared videos on the Hoop Tribe page were Rich Porter's first community of hoopers.

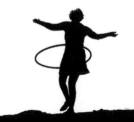

Facebook came along in 2006 with a much broader capacity. When Tribe.net became unstable and started to collapse, hoopers migrated en masse to Facebook. So many of them recreated their identities in that network that it immediately expanded a general awareness of hoopdance. For instance, people who had not been involved with the somewhat esoteric Tribe.net, but knew Rich Porter before he picked up the hoop, were introduced to hooping through Rich's Facebook page.

Philo Hagen's Hooping.org and SaFire's HoopCity.ca are key sites where hoopers connect. Both have forums, live chat, and private messaging. They allow members to upload videos, photos, and journals of their hooping process. When Jason Strauss (Jason Unbound) posted instructions on Hooping.org for making hoops, there was a rapid increase in the production of handmade hoops. HoopCity's Homestay Project helped hoopers find a host and a place to stay in any city they might be visiting, or to meet up in a particular location. Seattle's Wednesday Hoop Jam started that way.

Lynn Knickrehm-Fisher moderates the Northwest HoopGroup on Hooping.org. The hoops she and her friends played with in 1998 were the

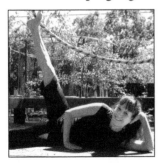

small plastic kind. "We brought our hoops everywhere, and even hooped as cow mascots (udders and all) for the local band Bovalexia (referring to a sudden urge to moo at cows)." Eventually she became the first certified hoopdance instructor in Idaho. In her video *Another Reason to Hula Hoop* she is cold, and a friend throws her a hoop. To prove how quickly she warms up, Lynn removes her winter jacket and sweater in mock burlesque, while waist hooping. Anytime you think it's too cold to hoop or you just want to raise your body temperature, start with warm layers to shed as you get moving. It won't take long.[16] [V]

Hooping without Borders

A search for hooping or particular hoopdancers on Vimeo or YouTube returns a mass of links. Lisa Lottie's 2008 video has had over three hundred thousand views and has been a major inspiration to hoopdancers around the world.[17] [V]

Lisa was living in Brighton, England, when a friend gave her a hoop to play with on the beach. That led to her background performance at the end of a fellow hoopdancer's video. Then she was offered a job traveling with a circus in India. "That's where it all went crazy! I guess you could say my hooping comes from traditional circus, because I learned all my tricks when I was living with the circus in India. Then I broke free to travel the world, living and teaching with my hoops, and performing along the way." London became a stopping place for Lisa because she could study for a degree in circus arts at the Circus Space school, train in her spare time, and street perform on the South Bank.

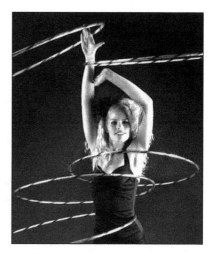

Gathering Abroad

Hoop teachers around the world travel to teach at hoopdance events outside their own culture. When Beth Lavinder (from the United States) met Gems Goddard (from the United Kingdom) at Hoopcamp in Santa Cruz, Gems invited Beth to teach at the U.K. Hoop Gathering that she organized in the rural location of Shropshire, England, called Wild Ways. It was Beth's first time in England, and Sue Wilkinson, organizer of the Hoop Club at the nearby Royal Leamington Spa, showed Beth the village before the weekend gathering of fifty-five people got started.

Beth taught two workshops and met a new breed of hoopdancers. "Brits are fresh and open to new ways of playing with the hoop. They have their own unique way of moving that is slightly different from mine, perhaps more influenced by traditional circus." They hooped and danced ecstatically together, and Chanti Hobbit and Emily Ball (the Pantaloonies) performed in their circus-influenced, endearing, and farcical British style.[18] V

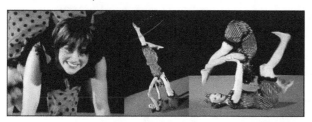

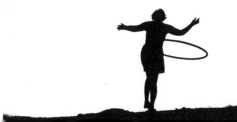

While Beth was at Wild Ways, she was invited to teach at Spin Matsuri, a three-day weekend of hoop, flow, and movement workshops held in October at the Seimei no Mori resort in Chiba, Japan. The location is an hour from Tokyo by train or car, and it was an opportunity for Beth to go back to a country she had lived in and loved. Between classes at Spin there were parties, breaks, and meal times in which participants from different cultures, who may or may not have spoken each other's language, became acquainted or reconnected with old friends.

Beth was scheduled to teach two one-and-a-half-hour outdoor classes, but at the appointed time it started to rain. She says, "It was the only rain we had, but it meant that I had to teach everyone at once indoors, and I was afraid a single class would be too large." The two classes were combined and held in the resort's gymnasium, which has a thirty-foot-high ceiling and a wall of curved glass that looks out at the smaller area of lush green lawn and trees where the classes would have been. Joining the two classes created a powerful energy that filled the space perfectly.

Beth's teaching style is modeled on Baxter's HoopPath. She started with a review of the basic concepts of hooping. Then she led her class to move about blindfolded. And finally, she taught various hooping techniques. In most classes visual demonstration would be enough to convey necessary information for hoopdancing, but the HoopPath method relies on metaphors that require language. Beth found it difficult to teach in two languages at the same time. "I got the information across by explaining some of the concepts in Japanese and some in English. In demonstrations I spoke slowly in English and inserted some Japanese words, which worked out well enough." She and the retreat staff worked hard to ensure good crossover in communication. It was important to Beth that the people whose country she was in did not feel excluded.

When the Wham-O hoop came out in the 1950s, Japan banned it because the rotating hip action seemed indecent, but by 2009 the Los Angeles-based company Hoopnotica was shipping dance hoops to Japan fifty thousand at a time by container load. Japan's Hoop Lovers offered a "super chill" arm workout at the ocean's edge on Yuigahama Beach.[19] [V]

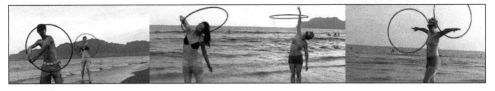

Manchester Hoop Congress

Gail O'Brien (Hoop Spin) hosted her own Hoop Congress in Manchester, England, after attending the U.K. Hoop Gathering. A sprightly yet pragmatic young woman from Northern Ireland, Gail stands five feet tall, is full figured, and is tenacious about practicing. When she started hoopdancing in 2008, she thought it might be a good way to lose weight, but she says, "That quickly went out the window. For me, and many others, the train- 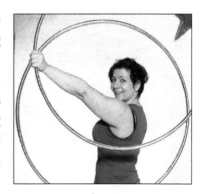 ings given by Christabel Zamor and Diana Lopez were a way for us to meet up because we were scattered all around the country" The result? More U.K. hoop stars.[20] [V]

As hoopdance became more important to Gail, she attended Hoopcamp and Harbin Hoop Jam in the United States. "We were still new to hooping in the U.K., and the playing field was level. Whereas in the U.S., a hierarchy of teachers and students had been developed. The jam is the way we play in Europe. We are also more cynical. On stage we expect to get heckled. If someone messes up, we would be hollering 'Do it again, only better!' In the U.S. everyone would clap and be supportive."

Hoopdancing professionally was the furthest thing from Gail's mind when she began to play with hoops. She had a secure position as a physiotherapist with a pension and good career prospects. Then one year the festival season started right after she was promoted in her job. She had offers to perform and travel, but her request to work part-time was denied. A week later she quit the job and gave away everything that didn't fit in her rucksack. She was freed up for teaching and learning—at SWHoop with Emma Kerr, in Thailand with the Spark Circus, or in Bali with Jaguar Mary. Gail says with mock contempt, "Life is so hard since I gave up my job."

Working in physiotherapy, Gail had provided hands-on healing through England's National Health Service. Now the women who come

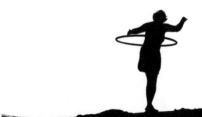

to her hoopdance classes take a positive attitude home with them. So, "no," she says, "I don't regret my decision to leave steady employment behind." As she builds her new career in hooping, her contribution to society is inspirational.[21] V

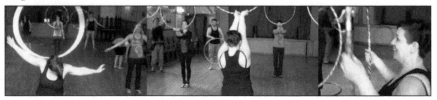

Gail was raised to go to school and then secure a nine-to-five job, but her parents approved of Gail doing the thing she loved. When she bought them a round-trip ticket to the United States, they planned to tour around for three months to see what their daughter was up to. With her own version of "chest hooping," Gail was a star in the firmament of the 2011 Colorado Spin Summit, a Rocky Mountain retreat.[22] V

SWHoop

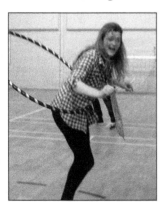

SWHoop is a hoop gathering presented by Emma Kerr of Hooping Mad in the southwest of England. Emma has drawn together more than two hundred hoopers in her home city of Bristol alone. Hooping Mad also offers classes in Bath, Cheltenham, and South Wales, as well as touring workshops throughout the year and two-day hooping retreats in summer.

Emma originally picked up hooping at a festival. She was supposed to be teaching *poi* workshops, but everyone seemed more interested in the hooping, so she decided to join them and was given her first adult-sized hoop. She had been studying for a PhD in immunology at the time and was working long hours in the lab. "I was short on cash, lived in student accommodations acting as a warden for a hundred and twenty undergraduate students, and spent many evenings in the hall 'on call,' which meant I had loads of time to practice hoopdance and to pore over video tutorials."

Emma's first opportunity to earn money from hooping came when a colleague asked her to teach a belly-dance workshop at an international youth summer camp. "I laughed," she says, "because I'm *rubbish* at belly dancing, but I suggested that I might come and teach hooping." She made a slew of blank hoops and spent a day helping young people from all over the world decorate them. Then she taught them tricks. From there she became a regular teacher at youth clubs and started teaching hoop classes while writing her doctoral thesis. Within months she had four weekly classes in the center and south of Bristol.

When Emma took her first workshop with Sharna Rose, England's premiere hoopdancer, she was star-struck and completely intimidated—so much so that she ran away before the class ended. By the following summer she had gained confidence and made many hoop friends, including Sharna, Beth Lavinder, Gail O'Brien, and the Pantaloonies. She was invited to join the Travelling Light Circus and jumped at the chance.

Emma's boss, family, and friends were in shock when, after completing her doctorate and six months of postdoctoral work, she decided to teach hooping full time. She increased the number of classes she was teaching, enlisted her best students to become teachers, and codesigned a hooping class for mothers. She also began spending more time with Bristol's circus hoopers, whose work she valued, though it was little known in the hoop-dance community.

Emma specializes in twin hooping; she and Steve Bags are so smooth that just watching pushed my own meager attempts to a new level.[23] [V]

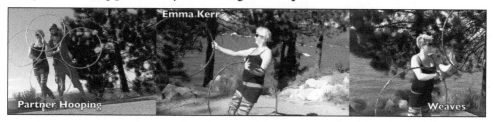

Emma Kerr
Partner Hooping   Weaves

England can be beautiful in the summer, but it gets cold in October. Emma organized SWHoop to break up the winter hooping lull, when the rain increases and hoopers are forced into cramped living rooms. The first SWHoop shied away from performance to focus on flow. In the second, American hoopers Baxter, Beth, and Brecken taught with the homegrown talents of the Pantaloonies, Sharna, Gail, and Bags. SWHoop's lineup for

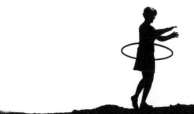

the third year created a hoop fusion, with workshops in contemporary hoopdance, circus hooping, American Indian hoop dance, and rhythmic gymnastics.

Sacred Journeys

There is a great deal of accomplished, athletic hoopdancing that goes on around the globe in meet-ups and in video. But the goal of the hoopdance revolution is not solely about expertise. Jaguar Mary (Ja Má) cofounded the DC Hoop Collective in Washington, D.C., and hoopdance is her tool

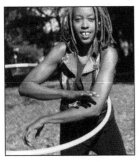

"for transformation on this planet." In her process of learning, dropping the hoop is an inspiration rather than a defeat, and she readily dreams of dancing in ways that her body is not actually able to understand—quite yet. Through persistent, conscientious practice, she moves toward an intention to flow without hurry. "I continue to apply myself, develop skill, and become more aware. The practice is forever." [24] [V]

Ja Má organizes Sacred Circularities retreats that function as a laboratory for the intermingling of intentional hoopdance with meditation, sound play, and yoga. Each group supports the individual quests of its members. "We travel to sacred places to send out waves of love. We assist, amplify, and anchor the planet's vibration through ecstatic movement by embracing our own divinity in hoopdance. We spin to replicate the movement of planets and stars. We visit ancient sites of significant spiritual vibration to acknowledge our roots. And we pray together in gratitude for the brilliance of life. Flow is the way we change. The fire of transformation and the interplay of life and death are the eternal spin we are in."

Ja Má has over twenty-five years of movement experience, and a master of fine arts degree. New York's Museum of Modern Art and biennials of contemporary art around the world show her films. Her interview videos document the hoopdance movement. As a healer she is certified in massage and Reiki therapy. When she moves the hoop around her own body—throwing it, catching it, jumping through it—hooping is play, dance, and meditation all twirled into one joy-inducing activity. "I sit and meditate, or I hoop—both open my mind. As corny and old school as it sounds: hooping is mind blowing."

Chapter Seven Links

www.HoopDanceBook.com/chapter7

1. *The 1st Burning Man.* Oct. 9, 2008.

2. *BurningMan 2004.* Feb. 16, 2007.

3. *Hoop Convergence 2010.* May 27, 2010.

4. *Miss Saturn: Hula Hoop Artiste.* Jan. 27, 2008.

5. *FlowShow2: Unexpected Progressions.* Apr. 30, 2010.

6. *Movement Play Official Trailer.* Apr. 2, 2010.

7. *Contact Improvisation at Luminz Studio.* Jan. 16, 2008.

8. *Rich Porter & Tropo @ Movement Play 09.* Aug. 9, 2009.

9. *Hoop Camp 2009.* Oct. 2, 2009.

10. *Harbin Hoop Jam.* Dec. 6, 2008.

11. *Hoop Tutorial Jo's Legocopter.* Mar. 6, 2011.

12. *Infinite Patterns.* Oct. 23, 2010.

13. *Yes We Can.* Jan. 14, 2009.

14. *Bay Area Hoopers—Jan 15, 2012.* Jan. 15, 2012.

15. *How to Hula Hoop Rap Song.* Jul. 5, 2011.

16. *Another Reason to Hula Hoop.* Jul. 23, 2009.

17. *Hula Hoop Dancer—Lisa Lottie.* Jul. 27, 2008.

18. *The Pantaloonies.* Dec. 22, 2009.

19. *Super Chill Arm Workout.* Aug. 4, 2009.

20. *UK Hoop Stars.* Jul. 15, 2010.

21. *Gail O'Brien (Hoop Spin) Hoop Workshops in Bristol—May 2011.* May 4, 2011.

22. *Spin Summit 2011.* Jul. 26, 2011.

23. *Bags and Emma's Twin Hooping Weekender.* Sep. 8, 2011.

24. *It's a Practice: Jaguar Mary Hoops.* Feb. 13, 2012.

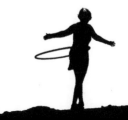

PART III

Hoopdance

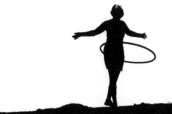

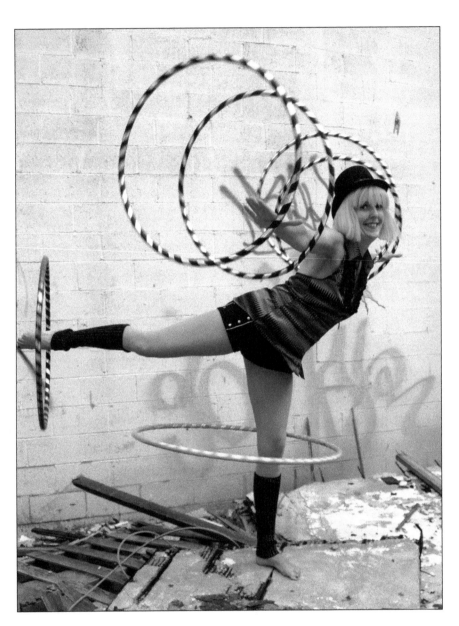

Revolva performing with six hoops

EIGHT

History and Performance

The past does not repeat itself, but it rhymes.
—Mark Twain, author and humorist

After taking classes, practicing, and meeting hoop stars, I still had gaps in my understanding of the history of hoopdancing. In 2009 no one seemed to know where the idea for big dance hoops came from. I started a deeper investigation with Judith Lanigan's charming and informative book *The Hula Hoop* and discovered a rich tradition in the circus and vaudeville. During the twentieth century circus acts developed the use of hooping in Russia, Australia, and China. Jugglers spun hoops on parts of their bodies, and hoop rolling was integrated into rhythmic gymnastic routines, but none of these were dance hoops.

Next I heard about Beth Childers. She had been a friend of the String Cheese Incident band when hooping champion Paul Blair made her a large-size hoop. She brought it to a SCI show for dancing, and Paul made more hoops for the band to give away. Learning that Paul had made the first hoop satisfied my curiosity for a while; but after I saw a video in which Mat Plendl used a very large hoop well before anyone had heard of String Cheese Incident, I was determined to keep digging.[1] V

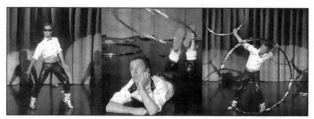

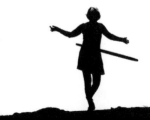

The Advent of Plastic

Betty Shurin (Betty Hoops) directed me to Bill Hess, whose father had been a chemist and industrial engineer. Before his death, William Hess Sr. owned a company that produced plastic pipe and fittings. I drove down to Santa Barbara to meet his son, Bill Jr. He told me that in 1954 his father had taken him and his sister to Goldwater's department store in downtown Tucson, Arizona, to see American Indian hoop dancers.

Impressed by the dances, Hess Sr. made hoops for his children from the tubing he manufactured. He then tried to market his hoops to the big toy companies without success. Two years later George Jennings, a plastics maker who had a factory in Australia, came to visit. Jennings wanted to learn about making plastic pipe for irrigation. When he saw bare plastic hoops hanging on the Hess office wall, he asked about them. Bill Jr. demonstrated. Jennings had seen the wooden hoops used in gym classes in Australia and thought he might be able to market a plastic replacement. Within six months of his return home, he is said to have sold five hundred thousand plastic hoops.

In the meantime, Spud Melin had cofounded the Wham-O Manufacturing Company with Richard Knerr in a garage in South Pasadena, California. Melin saw the plastic hoops Jennings made in Australia and came back to California, engaging the Hess factory to make hoops from extruded Marlex pipe for Wham-O. Bill Jr. says, "Spud Melin became a

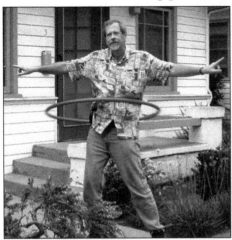

family friend. He was great at marketing and advertising. When he announced his hoop, everybody wanted one. About four cents' worth of materials and a few cents of labor went into a hoop that sold for around $1.98."

Bill Sr. manufactured Wham-O hoops in a variety of sizes with colorful stripes, but his son was probably the first person to have used a plain black irrigation-tubing hoop. Bill Jr. has been hula hooping since 1955.

The World's Greatest Hooper

In 1987 Mat Plendl appeared on the Johnny Carson show with an over-sized hoop and was dubbed "The World's Greatest Hula Hoop Artist." He

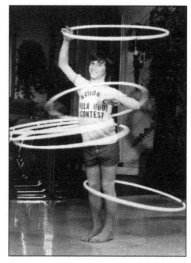

had been U.S. National Hula Hoop Champion at the age of thirteen, and at twenty-four he performed his hoop act on Johnny Carson's *Tonight Show* three times in six months. He's been dazzling audiences around the globe ever since. I visited Mat in his dressing room at Teatro ZinZanni in San Francisco, where he performs in shows that feature comedy, song and dance, juggling, and aerial arts. He told me he has been hula hooping since he was ten years old.

In 1972 Mary Howe sat next to Mat in the fourth grade. "I followed Mary around like a puppy, I did everything she did, and we had many extracurricular activities in common. We drew, took drum lessons, and played tetherball." When Mary asked Mat if he wanted to go to a hula-hooping contest, of course he did. "I surprised myself that I could do it, and I entered the local qualifying round for the U.S. national competition." He made it to both city and state trials, and after just three months of practice he placed third in the far west regional finals. Mary got first place and went to the nationals, which were held at Universal Studios. She won second place. Mat was in the audience because he lived nearby, and he was inspired. He thought, "I'm going to win this whole thing." It took three more years for him to reach that goal and win the city, state, and regional contests.

Semifinals for the national competition required five compulsory moves, performed for fifteen seconds each. They were simple things: hooping around the knees, standing on one leg, getting the hoop from the knees to the waist and back, getting it to go from the knees to the neck and back down, and the "hula hop" or "footsy," in which the hoop is hopped over as it rotates around one ankle.

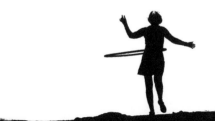

Hooping around the waist was not one of the trials, but in the freestyle set to music Mat could do whatever he wanted. He choreographed his routine to the theme from *SWAT,* edgy stuff for a preteen when other youngsters were performing to standards like "Tijuana Taxi." Most competitors in the national hula hooping championships were young women, but in 1975 both finalists were young men. The championships were televised on the *Dinah Shore Show,* and Mat won the whole thing.[2] V

As a youth Mat had performed with the Redondo Beach community theater, in which kids got lead parts in the children's theater and small parts in the adult civic light opera. He continued acting in high school and developed a love-hate relationship with the hoop. "No one wants to be defined by one thing, especially a young person who is ambitious, talented, and wants to be creative." In college he studied musical theater, and he rarely did anything with hoops.

Mat was working as an insurance salesman when he moved to Los Angeles to pursue an acting career. He had vowed to a friend that he would go to two auditions per week, and time was running out when he came upon a casting call flyer from the Variety Arts Center, a downtown Los Angeles theater that had hosted some of the biggest names in entertainment since the 1920s. He brought his hoops to the audition. "The judges liked my demonstration but wanted more of an act. I saw a giant roll of tubing coiled up against the back wall of the theater, and that gave me the idea to add a large hoop." Mat's act was accepted when he parodied the characters in the movie *Chariots of Fire,* exaggerating the ultra-slow motion of his six-foot-diameter hoop to the movie's dramatic theme song.

Harry Anderson, star of the popular TV situation comedy *Night Court,* hosted the last two weeks of the Variety Arts Center show. Mat says, "We got so much attention that most of the acts were picked up for the *Merv Griffin Show* or the *Tonight Show* with Johnny Carson." Mat was somewhat embarrassed by his hula-hooping act, but there was a guest hosting for Johnny the night he was booked, so he thought, "Nobody's going to watch this." The next day he had fifteen job offers and was signed by an agent for comedians. A six-city tour with Oldsmobile and various other contracts resulted from that appearance, and Carson booked him again for New Year's Eve. That one show launched his career. Then in Canada he was signed by an international agent and traveled to Europe, South America, and Japan.

Collision of Then and Now

When Mat won the hula-hooping championship in 1975, there were one and a half million youth participating in competitions nationwide. It was well before Burning Man, but contestants worked hard with small hoops to develop hooping as a performance art. They experimented with music and were judged critically on continuity, degree of difficulty, and show-manship. As contemporary hoopdancers created more complex routines, they needed to use smaller, lighter hoops.

"I could have told them that." Mat says. "I was doing it before most of them were born." His career had started in the last days of showbiz, when variety performance was a staple on broadcast television. TV was how he became known. There was no link to check out his video then. He sent VHS cassettes in the mail. In 2002 Mat came home to Teatro ZinZanni. It brought together everything he does: theater, music, comedy, costumes, lighting, and the big finale hula-hooping act. It wasn't always so, but via the Internet you can now see Mat practice on the Teatro ZinZanni stage.[3] V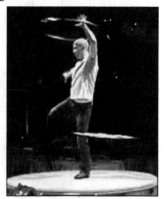

ZinZanni's antique *spiegeltent,* constructed in wood and canvas and decorated with mirrors and stained glass, opened in San Francisco on Pier 29, along the city's Embarcadero, in 2000. As a dinner theater, its shows play to local residents, tourists, and corporate parties. Patty Duke saw Mat there when she was doing *Wicked* downtown and had a Sunday night off. When actors come in, Mat gets excited. "They appreciate everything we do. The other extreme would be a room filled with lawyers and engineers who may not respond at all. That's a hard group to play to."

Integrating cirque-style performance with the serving of food, and working interactively with an audience of three hundred people seated 360 degrees around the stage, take a high level of energy and awareness.

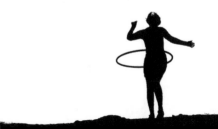

Each performer has to be in a specific place at every moment of the three-and-a-half-hour show. Wait staff, crew, performers, and audience members are all mixed together. Mat considers every performance a minor miracle. "The audience at Teatro is not just 'out there.' A waiter could be summoned to a table during a transition, or someone could head for the restroom just when a new act is coming down the same aisle. We've got to have our radar up for every little thing that goes on in that room." It is an intimate situation, but Mat performed as a youngster on the Santa Monica pier for passersby, so he has never been afraid to look into the faces of his audience in close proximity.

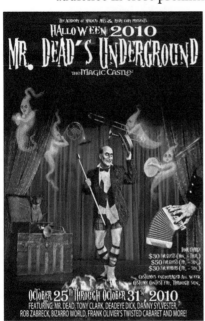

Over the course of thirty years, Mat has developed multimedia performance pieces that incorporate storytelling, projected visuals, bizarre characters, and theremin music, eerie electronic sounds from an instrument that is controlled by the player's hands without touching it. These talents culminated in his one-man show, *Mr. Dead's Underground,* which premiered in Los Angeles in 2010. Mr. Dead, a singing and dancing corpse, was partly inspired by Mat's father who suffered from Alzheimer's disease before his death. Mat says, "Mr. Dead is endearingly dead, not like a flesh-eating zombie. His foot is taped on. It falls off, he sticks it back on, and when he hoops at the end, the crowd goes wild."

Dizzy with Hoops

Before he discovered irrigation tubing, Paul Blair (Dizzy Hips) used toy hoops to dance at music concerts, hooping and performing tricks like getting down on the floor to spin the hoop around a raised foot. A 1991 Phish concert at Evergreen State College in Olympia, Washington, was the first show he brought hoops to for dancing. Later, working on a construction job in Colorado gave him the opportunity to make a larger version for String Cheese Incident. Paul says, "The first hoopers were Annie Dugan, myself, and Betty Hoops, and later, Anah Reichenbach. Anyone who says it started in Los Angeles, San Francisco, or especially New York (way later) is full of Marlex—the worst kind of plastic for making a hoop."

Paul believes that Mat Plendl has the best five-minute hooping act in the world. Among hoopdancers he particularly admires Revolva, a performer from Detroit who is more theatrical than many he has seen. He says, "Revolva's act builds to a climax with a beginning, a middle, and an end."

- Beginning sets a mood and introduces the hoop.
- Middle grows in intensity and speed.
- End pulls out all the stops with a grand finale.

In order to perform Paul had to confront his fears. Fear stops the creative process. It blocks energy pathways and changes the body's chemistry. At seventeen he had tried an experiment to see if he could have fun without drinking or doing drugs. "It was kind of lonely. I don't think I could have done it without something like hula hooping as an icebreaker. The hoop gave me a reason to be at the party." At first he experienced extreme discomfort, and his heart rate spiked temporarily. But after a while showing off became a buffer. He could pretend no one was watching, and the audience could also pretend they were not watching. In a performance the relationship is different: the performer and the audience acknowledge that the show is going on. After getting past his fear, he had to get past the buffer in order to perform on an actual stage in front of people. "When I finally did," he says, "I was energized by the two-way connection."

Juggling and even a lasso have made their way into Paul's acts. He took up the lasso in order to do a trick called "the wedding ring," in which he twirls a rodeo lasso around his wiry figure, as he hoops inside it. For him, flow is the building block between each trick. "The difference between hooping performance and hoopdancing is that flow is *hidden* in performance tricks. They are so impressive that you don't notice flow; like when Mat Plendl catches the hoop on his foot and throws it around his neck in 0.75 seconds to get to the beginning of the next big trick."

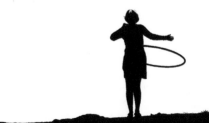

When Paul was a dance major in college, doing dance routines while hula hooping eliminated him from most studio classes. He is a rebel. "If you are an adult and you go skipping down the street, that's rebellious. Add a hoop, and it gets even better." He thought it was cheating when Anah used her hands to revolve the hoop around her ankles and legs, transferring it from one hand to the other to bring it up the core of her body. On second thought he concluded, "I could see that using hands and arms in the dance looked good. If it looks good, who can complain?" When Paul traverses the playground rings hand over hand while waist hooping, he's a happy Spider Man.[4] V

What keeps Paul interested in hooping is problem solving. If he wakes up in the middle of the night thinking of a new trick, he has to do it. He started two-person "tandem" hooping in 1993 when he had a crush on a young woman. He looked at her, and then at his two hoops: separation. How would he get close? "Then a light went off in my brain. I took the two hoops apart, joined them as one, and we hooped together."

Tandem hooping can be riotous fun between people who don't mind getting close, because two bodies have to move as one within the same hoop. The easiest way to start is with one person behind the other, both facing the same direction and moving as if stuck with glue from chest to hips. You can also try it face to face. The Twistin Vixens, Colleen and Kayla, from St. Cloud, Minnesota dance in tandem back to back.[5] V

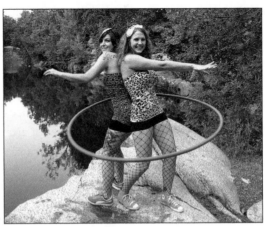

Paul takes his hoops everywhere. When he performed in Dubai, he found that most things there were privately owned. "Shopping malls are their equivalent of our parks, and I performed there three hours a day, six days a week, plus setup and breakdown time. It's hard work, but they pay well, treat you well, and the food is great."

Clowning for Life

Annie Dugan is an artist with a master's degree in physical theater. Circus trained, she was never part of the jam band scene. She worked in circuses in the United States from 1993 to 1995. "I started clowning in San Francisco as Ms. Ginger Snappe, was the first hula-hooping street performer in the Bay Area, and the only woman in North America performing with hoops at street festivals."

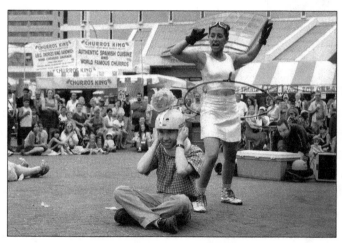

Annie went on to become the artistic director of Firefly Theatre and Circus in Edmonton, Alberta. Together with John Ullyatt, the troupe combined the visceral experience of circus arts with the emotional experience of theatre. Annie says, "Our stories take place on the ground and in the air; we play inside theatres, outside at roadway intersections, and suspended from buildings." Annie and Lyne Gosselin created an acrobatic hula-hooping routine in which Annie balances on Lyne's shoulders, stomach, and feet while hooping to the gasps and laughs of the audience. Firefly

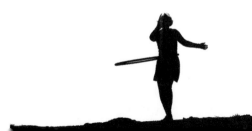

Theatre established Alberta's first aerial arts program, offering classes to the public and workshops to professional artists.

Judith Lanigan (Miss Judy) is an Australian entertainer who has performed in nightclubs, art festivals, and street theater all over the world. Spinning as many as thirty hoops at once around various parts of her body, she is recognized by Austrade (the Australian Trade Commission) as an official

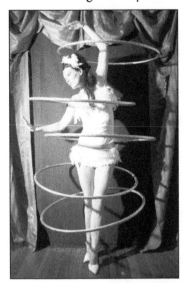

national export. She studied magic with Barcelona's veteran magician Andreu Sabadell and clowning with Brazil's Angela de Castro, who reclaimed theatre clowning as a modern art form in 1986. She discovered hooping while training in trapeze at Moscow Circus School, the world's oldest circus school, which had trained only young athletic Russians from 1927 until after the fall of communism.

Miss Judy calls her approach to performing "clownthink," and her sense of play is equal to her ability for drama. She combines a unique brand of farce with proficient, graceful movement in an act based on *The Dying Swan*. At the Theatre Royal during the Castlemaine State Festival in 2009, she gave an enchanting hoopdance rendition of the ballet that had been choreographed for Anna Pavlova in the early twentieth century. Accompanied by Heraldo and his Flaming Flamingo Orchestra, Miss Judy deftly spun her way through the dance. Then she twirled multiple hoops, frantically adding more as they were flung at her from the sidelines of the stage until, as the ballet demands, the swan dies, collapsing into the splits, the back of a limp hand raised to her brow as the lights go down.[6] V

Gender Bending

Karis Wilde (Karis) is an American performance artist who, in a video ad for a European electric razor, tells us that around the age of seven his mom caught him wearing her makeup. When I picked him up at the Oakland airport, he was even lovelier than his image on film.[7] V

Eager to catch up with friends in San Francisco, Karis told me his story as we drove over the Bay Bridge. He was born in Mexico but grew up in Los Angeles, and "fitting in" has always been his biggest struggle. "First I tried being more masculine, but I wasn't happy with myself. I tried being more feminine because I felt that I should be, but 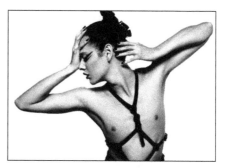 no, I am somewhere in the middle. I have always been androgynous, but I thought that when I was older, I would be accepted. Instead I found that most people don't think outside the box. Even in the gay world there are many limitations; it's just a different box."

On his eighteenth birthday Karis threw a pool party in Los Angeles. One of his girlfriends brought a hoop. He loved it, and she gave him one. He took it to another friend's barbecue, where a belly dancer saw him hooping and invited him to be in her show. Karis says, "I never had business cards or promoted myself, but after that I got bookings." He was performing in both Los Angeles and New York before he discovered Burning Man, where he met other hoopers. "It was strange to find a whole world I knew nothing about that was right here all the time."[8] V

No matter where he is Karis likes wearing women's clothing, and he doesn't mind being called "she." Experimenting with the "Victor-Victoria" paradigm in a burlesque act, he proved that he is equally beautiful in either gender: she comes on stage to wild cheers and catcalls from the audience as a sexy woman. "Then I strip off the top of my costume, switch over to being a boy, and bring out the hoop. Gender identification no longer matters: sexy as a woman, sexy as a man." His costumes are as elaborate and glamorous as his hooping is perfectly crafted. Finding the right balance is a fine art. "If I am wearing a wig and high heels, I don't cross over into drag-queen territory. As a man I embrace my masculine side." The more makeup she wears, the stronger and more controlled is her hooping. When his appearance is masculine, his hooping becomes all the more sensual.

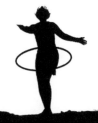

As an entertainer he believes in giving people something spectacular for their time, attention, and money. "At the end of the day," he says, "the most important thing is to use my talent to make people think."

His friend Tiffany was inspired to give Karis his name, which means grace, love, and mercy, because those were the qualities that she saw in him. "My stage name was born out of something deeply beautiful," he reflects, "and it reaches into even the most superficial parts of my life to keep me grounded. I love putting on my costumes and going on stage, but that is largely fantasy. When I hear my name announced before I go out there, it reminds me of who I really am." That allows him to bring his authentic self to hoopdancing, whether it is for an extravagant exhibition or a solo dance to a simple drum beat.[9] [V]

Motown Girl

Kari Jones (Revolva), one of Paul Blair's favorite hoopdancers, admits to being so far gone into vaudeville land that her experience of hoopdance might be uncommon. Still, she is a major figure in the movement, performing professionally with hoops since 2002 in Detroit. By 2010 she was teaching at hoop gatherings and working in circus shows across the country. She cofounded Circus Artemis in Portland, Oregon, and is a first-generation contemporary hoopdancer. Revolva is out to prove that "Funny *is* sexy!" and the hoop is her platform.

In mini plays Revolva might depict a jilted bride or a space explorer, setting up a dilemma and then bursting into hoopdance, continuing the story with gestures and facial expressions while she spins. "As an introvert it is freeing to embody a persona through language, theatrics, or dance." Her hooping performance and videos come from a love of storytelling. *The Revolvies Pre-Show 2011* is an example of her talent and playfulness. Revolva leads the 99 percent to take back hooping awards from the 1 percent. It's Occupy Hoopdance. (Includes a hoopoff with Spiral) [10] [V]

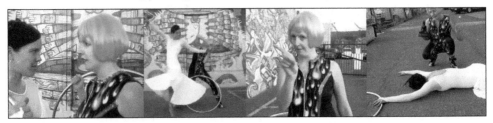

In preschool Kari went to dance classes, at nine she began performing in community theatre, and in high school she had leading roles in plays and studied jazz dance and ballet. Because dancing was the thing that made her feel the most centered as a teenager, her parents moved their car out of the garage to give her space to practice. "I'd go out there with my cassette player to stretch and dance, even in the freezing Michigan winter."

Kari studied creative writing and began combining monologue with dance for solo performances at the University of Michigan. Later, working as an advertising copywriter, she found herself on stage with hoops and an alter ego. A friend was directing the Pangea Experience, a Detroit arts collective that included several musicians and artists who were also actors. Her Revolva persona was invited to perform with them.

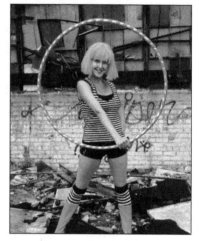

Revolva was born in Motown, a city with a vibrant music scene and legendary music history. Detroit techno has influenced house music internationally. Even so, Revolva was working harder for national recognition than she might have had to do if she were on either coast. The Internet changed that. When she discovered hooping on Tribe.net and YouTube, she shouted to her roommate, "Get in here and look at the computer! I found my family!" She met other Midwest hoopers online, and Chicago's KC Mendicino made Revolva's first fire hoop.

By 2004, Revolva was a performance machine. She joined the burlesque troupe Hell's Belles Girlie Revue and performed with them at the 2500 Club, a place that was so small they had to get ready for the show in the kitchen. "It was actually great to be smooshed in there with all the burly girls. I learned many makeup tricks from them." In one year Revolva went from playing on small stages, where her hoops couldn't help but hit a guitar player, to big venues like the Emerald Theater and the Masonic Temple.

The Detroit Roller Derby originally hired her as a cheerleader, but Julie Hecker, who passed away in 2010, was in charge of the squad. She gave

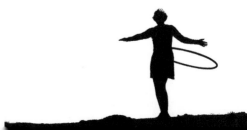

Revolva a spot in the halftime show. It was a solo hit. She twirled her hoops acrobatically for the second-period intermission as well, and did it for every bout until she moved to Oregon.

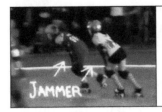

Detroit Derby Girls, founded in 2005, is a women's flat-track roller derby league—women power that is making a difference in the community.[11] [V]

Hoopdancers are bound to one another through their common reverence for the hoop regardless of geography or style. From Oregon, Revolva helped plan the first Hoop Convergence in North Carolina. "When your body, mind, and spirit have been transformed through this particular form of dance, it doesn't take any effort at all to connect with someone else who knows how that feels. It was exciting to dream about a convergence online and then actually see it come to fruition. Now I can't imagine going through life without my hooping friends."

Revolva's version of hoopdance is seriously funny. Whether she is dressed in a flamboyant pink wig or demure black leotard, she is always clowning to get her message across. On the streets and on stage she jumps through flaming hoops as if the danger were an afterthought. Her characters range from outrageous to flirtatious. And when she encounters promoters who just want to see a woman in very little clothing, she tells them, "That's not what I do." Often she is able to reset their expectations, dancing with multiple hoops and props in a variety of roles that are sexy, modest, and powerful. (See Kari Jones (Revolva) in resources.)

Revolva is a power name. People laugh and ask her, "Do you know that sounds like a female body part?" That's partly the reason she chose it. "My name embodies the concept of spiraling, and it speaks to key aspects of my personality: Detroit Rock City girl, feminist, creator of new words, and devotee of spinning arts. The hoop is my weapon—for creating rather than destroying. It goes beyond business; it's spiritual." In mid-career, Revolva shares the stage with well-known vaudeville acts. Sometimes she's the only woman in the lineup doing comedy and talking on stage. At Circus Artemis in Portland, where strength and skill ruled, technicians and performers were women, and Revolva played to a full house.

Inspiring people to be themselves is Revolva's goal, and she uses the hoop to foster centeredness. "I want girls and women to know that there is more than one way to be themselves. Whatever they want to make it, they can be funny, smart, loud, and sassy." Touring with New Old Time Chautauqua, she performed a duet stage act with Vanessa Vortex for two and a half weeks. Between performances they made up routines to busk on the street for donations. Revolva says, "I look for support and inspiration from other female hoopers. People like Vanessa, Miss Saturn, and Alley 'Oop are right up my alley." 12 V

Chapter Eight Links

www.HoopDanceBook.com/chapter8

1. *Mat Plendl on the Johnny Carson Show.* 1987.

2. *Hula Hoop Mat Plendl Dinah Shore 1975.* Feb. 13, 2009.

3. *Hula Hoop Mat Plendl Hooping Rehearsal 2009.* Feb. 12, 2009.

4. *Spiderman? Monkey Man? No Hoopman!* Aug. 15, 2007.

5. *Tandem Hula Hooping.* Jun. 19, 2011.

6. *The Dying Swan & the FFO.* Apr. 13, 2009.

7. *Philips Satinelle Ice Epilator "Karis" Cannes Lions Award 2008.* Nov. 25, 2008.

8. *Karis @ Burning Man 2006.* Sep. 13, 2006.

9. *Karis.* Apr. 23, 2009.

10. *The Revolvies: 2011 Pre-Show.* Jan. 23, 2012.

11. *Detroit Derby Girls.* Jan. 29, 2009.

12. *Vanessa Vortex with the New Pickle Family Circus.* Jan. 28, 2010.

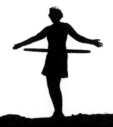

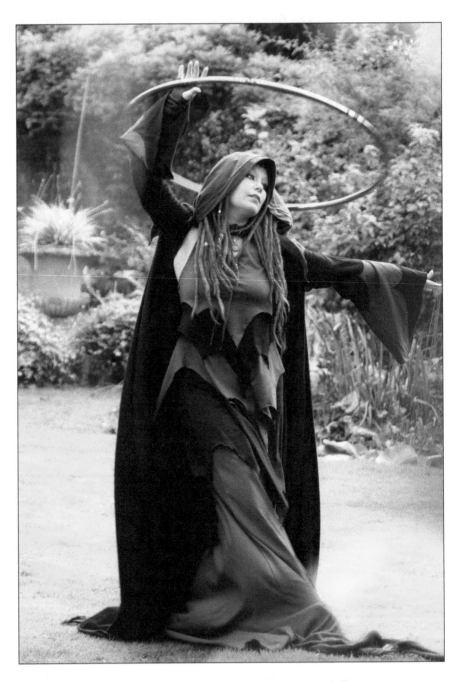

Frenchy wearing Le Nymph by Technodolly

NINE

Clothing, Hoops, and Music

Fashion has to do with ideas,
the way we live, what is happening.
—Coco Chanel, fashion designer

Whether on stage or in the park, hoopdancing calls for lifting and bending as well as swiveling and extending. Clothes that are stretchy and comfortable support maximum flexibility from head to toe. A glittering painted face adds to the fun, and the right shoes can help you slide with spectacular moves or keep your ankles and feet safe from falling hoops. Hoops can be decorated with tape that matches your ensemble, enhanced with rechargeable LED lights, or fitted with Kevlar wicks to be soaked in fuel and set afire. Music choices include everything that has a good beat, from tango to techno. What you wear, the hoop you choose, and the music you move to are all matters of personal choice.

What to Wear

Hoopdance outfits are a part of self-expression. While anything bulky or cumbersome, including big hair and jewelry, can inhibit the novice hooper, improbable outfits and accessories challenge skills with dramatic flare. You can wear street clothing, stretchy yoga clothes, a bathing suit, or nothing at all, but bare skin grabs a dance hoop best, and natural fibers cling well. Cotton and flax are excellent to start with. Tops without sleeves are best for successful shoulder hooping at any level of experience, as Caroleeena's tutorial points out.[1] V

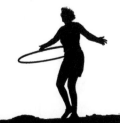

If you wear slippery fabrics, belts, or layers of loose clothing like sweaters and jackets, it gets more difficult. Stuff in your pockets, big hats, and uncomfortable footwear are also problematic, because it's hard to be creative if you are worried about revealing your body, losing things, or tripping over your own feet. Many hoopers take their shoes off right away, or wear yoga socks with non-slip rubber grips on the soles. For more protection you can wear dance shoes. Athletic shoes add support, but rubber soles can mark wooden studio floors and make spinning turns difficult.

Kacey Douglas, the traveling nurse we met in chapter 4, hoops for self-expression, and she performs as Miss Hoopstress. She considers fashion to be one of the draws of hooping. "You put your hoop on; it is part of your outfit. Whether you wear burlesque fluffy leg warmers, a tunic with points on the sleeves and a hood, or a rugged sexy leather getup, you stand out in the crowd."

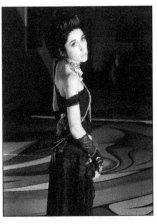

When Lauren Porter (Onyx) started hooping, she was married to Rich Porter, whom we met in chapter 3. She says, "Honestly, I think fashion and hooping have always been at odds. When you are learning, it's crucial to have the proper amount of grip between you and the hoop in order to feel what the hoop is actually doing. Because the connection of hoop to body is so important, hoopers are initially restricted in what they can wear." That said, Onyx turned to making clothes for her hoopdancing friends upon request. She describes her creations as "neo-Gothic, tribal, and very feminine."

Lauren's parents had tried unsuccessfully to get their young daughter to play team sports. "Why would I want to run and fight for a ball? All I wanted to do at recess was hoop." As soon as she was able to choose her own "sport," she chose dance. She danced in her room, in her yard, and in the grocery store waiting for her mom. Fifteen years later she was dancing in a very big hoop. "Rich helped me make a standing-to-above-the-belly-button hoop, and wrapped it in leather from skirts bought at thrift stores. Then we took it to the park. At first Rich sat on the sideline thinking hooping was for girls, but we all know how that turned out."

Onyx abandoned her large hoop for one that was dramatically smaller in 2007. "This changed everything. I began to spin, spin, spin, with tiny movements, lots of tricks, and quick variations of speed." Later she compromised with a somewhat larger but lighter hoop. Because it has less weight, she relies on the muscle memory she gained with her heavier hoop to predict where the lighter one is going to be. With the light hoop barely hanging on as it rotates, sagging and threatening to sweep the ground as it goes, she is transported, playing with her shadow or daydreaming of fantastic places where she can dress up every day.

Laura Blakeman (Shakti Sunfire) became a leader in the hoopdance movement as she traveled to teach and perform, but in college she followed the String Cheese Incident band. "The band and their community had much to do with shaping the hoopdancer I became. The crowd was decked out in clothes that were bright and colorful with rainbows, tutus, and hoops. It was almost like a circus."

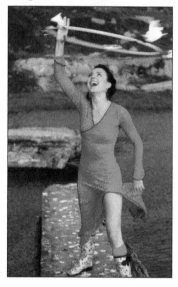

Costumes became so important to Shakti Sunfire that she began to make her own. She never learned "the right way," but sewing saved her money and gave her wardrobe a unique personality nonetheless. A friend taught her to make a pair of pants from a pattern. "It took me an entire night to figure it out, but once that first pair of pants was done, I could make anything." Her first costume, with a top made from a Colorado flag, was for a String Cheese Incident show in Las Vegas.

Starting with her mother's sewing machine, Shakti Sunfire bought her first industrial model in 2008. Good machines make sewing easier, and a serger, to finish seams and edges, opens up a world of creativity with stretchy fabric. Never having taken a class or had a teacher, she admits, "I do plenty wrong. I come up with an idea in my head or go to the fabric store to find something I like and feel I can work with, but the original

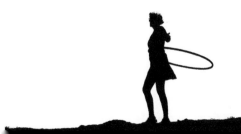

idea always evolves into something different." She doesn't follow logical steps from start to finish. Her process zigzags, swivels, and becomes an exploration of tie-dyed or shiny lamé for tops, white ruffles for the sides of flared pants, or a slit to the hips for a red dress. However she is dressed, her performance shines.[2] V

Clothing Designers

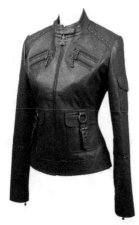

Mended Mosaic created a line of fashion clothing for hoopdancers that is burner friendly and fair trade, meaning that fire artists will love it and that it supports businesses in developing countries. KC Mendicino, pioneer of Chicago hoopdance, traveled the world with her husband, Louie, gathering inspiration from architecture, history, and people to create intricate designs that would be simple to wear. KC says, "We fused the romance and passion of old Spain, the debauchery of the 1920s, the hard-edged industrial age, and the dusty western saloon with formality from the Victorian era."

It started with the support of KC's parents when she came home from Australia and wanted to perform. "My mom sews, so she helped make my costumes. We would sit for hours sewing haphazard things without a pattern." When KC hooped in tandem with Christabel at Burning Man, they had dreadlocks and big fluffy boots to go with their blue-and-white bootie shorts. Halfway through the festival KC reverted to a black bikini, bandana, and fedora hat. "It felt earthy, like the desert playa. I could never get into the tropical hot pink, bright, and sunny costumes other hoopers seemed attracted to."

To be a cool hooper and still be herself, KC began making her costumes in the Burning Man style of leather and feathers. She made clothes she could wear while hooping or out on the town. Eventually people noticed and said, "I want a pair of those pants," or, "Would you make me that vest?" and she did. "A year later Louie and I had two investors. Together we started Mended Mosaic."

Ahni Radvanyi made the first pair of pants I purchased specifically for hoopdancing. We met at Hoopcamp in Santa Cruz, but Ahni's hoop journey started in Tampa. She was studying fashion design at the International Academy of Design and Technology in 2005 when she saw Alexis Nikitopoulos (Funkshine Hoop Troop) dancing with two hoops at a reggae festival. Ahni had never seen anyone defy gravity that way. "Alexis showed me how to do the walk through and the corkscrew as well as sustained spinning. Those became the first three things that I teach people."

Ahni's hoop mentor was Alexis Nikitopoulos of the Funkshine Hoop Troop in Tampa.[3]

Ahni follows what she loves, trusting that it will bring her to the right place, at the right time. At school she danced with her hoop between classes and met the people who connected her with fire hoopers and performance groups from other cities. Then she began teaching workshops and selling clothing at fire-spinning festivals around the country. In California she discovered AcroYoga and was invited to Seattle, where she engaged models and performers to create a postapocalyptic circus act for the Seattle Fashion Week runway.[4]

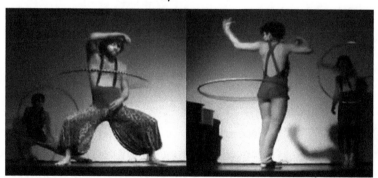

Ahni's reversible leather shorts, backless top with scarves and suspenders, and knee-high leggings gave her ample coverage while leaving plenty of bare skin for traction. For a duet she teamed up with Jon Coyne, author

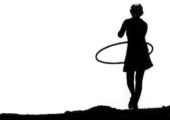

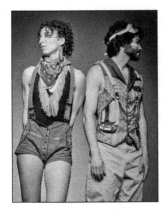

of the "How to Hoop" rap song. Jon's voluminous pantaloons accentuated his movements, leaving his feet free for spinning a hoop. High waists and suspenders link both outfits to traditional circus culture.

Ahni made Jon's pantaloons from a skirt she had worn in a previous phase of her life. "I enjoy 'up-cycling' as I like to call it—reusing fabric. For a vest Jon wore, I used silk, leather, and some bits and pieces of antique brass cabinet hardware that I collect." She makes reversible tops and bottoms, belts with optional pockets and attachable skirts, and shoulder holsters with pouches that zip on and off. Her clothing designs are modular because, she says, "Fortune favors the prepared and evolution favors adaptability."

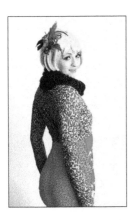

Annieland is Annie Weinert, whom I met at a workshop at Hoopcamp. Annie taught us how to make a recycled peephole costume top and shag armbands. She advises, "Don't allow your inner critic to compare yourself to other people. Everyone contributes something unique to the world that no one else can give." Her garments are playful and color-rich, often using materials salvaged from industrial scrap. She does all of her own design work, from pattern drafting to merchandising, and shares a "no-sew" idea with us. (See instructions at the end of the chapter.)

Dress Up Your Face

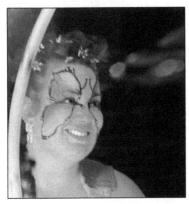

Face and body painting often complement hoopdance costuming simply because it's fun, it adds drama, or it enhances character. Toy stores and drugstore toy departments sell a variety of face-painting kits. If you are ready to go beyond the colorful line drawings offered to children at parties and fairs, professional supplies for face and body painting, and lots of instruction, can be easily found on the Internet. Isa Isaacs (GlitterGirl) offers a two-part tutorial.[5] Ⓥ

The Hoop You Choose

Nothing is more important to hoopdance than your hoop, whether the tubing is simply sanded for grip, inscribed with words, or covered in colorful tape. Making your own (see the end of chapter 2) can be a satisfying project, and hoop designers are continually perfecting the circles of largely negative space that we hoopdance within.

The Heart Sutra, one of Buddhism's best-known texts, teaches that form is emptiness and emptiness is form. The hoop is an empty circle. When Betty Shurin (Betty Hoops) lived at a yoga retreat in the early days of hoopdance, she wrote the entire Heart Sutra with permanent ink on the inner side of each hoop. They became prayer wheels, mandalas symbolizing the paradox of matter as nothingness. Later she designed a padded travel hoop that comes in segments. Using either five or six sections gives you two hoop sizes.

Laurie Hobbs, founder of Fluid Luminescence, uses her hoop to open clear channels of energy. "It's a tool that brings me to my center, connecting me with my body, my flow, my dance, and my source. When I pick up a hoop, I'm there. I'm present." She makes custom hoops with intentions inscribed on the tubing before it is wrapped in specialty tapes. Some people tell her what they want her to write, but more often her only instruction is to "write whatever you think I need." Laurie says, "It's a privilege to be an artist who makes things for other people. Even if the hoop stays 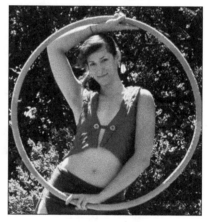 in someone's garage for a long time, there's a chance that it will one day become a tool of their self-knowing."

Hoop Training Wheels

When I went to San Luis Obispo to buy a hoop from Laurie, she had two in my size, each with different hidden words and colors of tape. The fiery

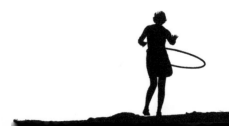

one in reds and orange was infused with intentions about coming up in the world and being outgoing. The one in watery blues and green was inspired by an inscription for going inward, getting in touch with emotions and peacefulness. I danced differently in each, even though they were of equal size and weight, and covered with the same type of tape. I kept coming back to the blue and green one because it *felt* right. Later, when I shared my hoops with a friend, she became so attached to the peacefulness of that hoop I passed it on to her.

Laurie began using foam, cork, and other nonslip tapes to cover her hoops after splitting her lip with a heavy slippery one, and noticing that some of the moves she knew she could do were impossible when she was wearing the wrong fabrics. She searched for grippier tapes that would help keep the hoop where you want it or that add padding for protection. Tackier tapes help you learn complex moves that require exactness in order to flow gracefully. They are gentler, and give you more wardrobe choices.

Tape that grips keeps the hoop in place the way training wheels help beginners keep a bike upright: Minimize pain. Maximize flow. Look great. Some hoopdancers think this is cheating, but Laurie wonders, "What is cheating? Are you in your flow, is the hoop moving, are you having fun? Is there a hoop manifesto somewhere that I forgot to read?"

Hoopdancers use Laurie's hoops to integrate moves that are "graceful and flowy" with "down-and-gritty chaos," entwining feminine and masculine energies. "When a woman uses her masculine energy to command the hoop, and when a man is able to integrate his grace in hooping, it just blows me away." If she feels a dry spell of inspiration coming on, she gets her "hoop juju" renewed by going to events where there is hooping and dancing going on every minute.

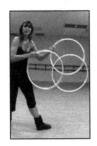

Laura Scarborough, founder of HoopCircle in Austin, Texas, designed another trainer—twenty-inch-diameter MagHoops. They add magical fun to hoop play by linking magnetically and separating easily in configurations of two, three, or four hoops. Laura explains that it's like having an extra pair of hands. In a trio set, two of the hoops have one magnet each, and the other has two, so that they can easily link in a chain without locking together.[6] [V]

A Grandfather's Influence

Jesica Flowers is a born entrepreneur. Even as a teenager she had a tie-dyed T-shirt company that did well. "I'm always running my own something, and hooping helps me keep my sanity." She won a who-can-hula-hoop-the-longest contest in fourth grade and did all the standard moves back then. At Burning Man in 1999, she saw a handful of hoopers. "Wait a minute," she realized. "Those are like my Grandpa's hoop." Then somebody asked her, "Hey, do you know how to make these bigger hoops?" and Jesica went into business again.

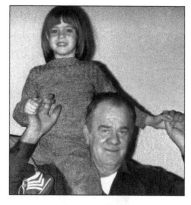

Jesica liked to hoop while watching TV in the early 1980s, but her toy hoops had balls inside them that clacked and made it hard to concentrate. She turned to a plumber, who loved tinkering in his workshop, for a solution. "My grandfather Wallace Marquess, who I called Wallygator, made my first custom hoop. Years later I was tempted to decorate it, but Wallygator's hoop remains blank with just a little piece of electrical tape where he applied it at the connection point."

Compared to what her thrifty grandmother Carolyn Marquess had taught her, the early dance hoops seemed expensive. "Large hoops were going for at least thirty-nine dollars plus shipping. I didn't think everyone would be able to pay that, so I decided to make an affordable option for people as frugal as my Nana." In first-generation hooper style, she and her helpers do all their production in-house, pulling back on advertising when they need to catch up with fulfilling orders. YourHoop offers the standard hoop sizes with custom color combinations as well as mini pairs, tandem hoops, and collapsible ones.

Coil It Down and Go

Before Diana Lopez, founder of BodyHoops, created the collapsible Infinity Travel Hoop, she was a sixth-grade teacher. When surgery ruled out her

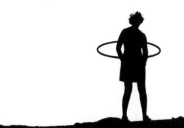

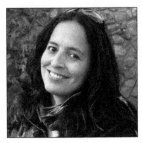

usual exercise for a few months, she hoopdanced just to keep moving. It was so helpful to her own healing process that she added hooping to her students' curriculum. She also started making a lot of hoops. After hand-wrapping hundreds of them between 2001 and 2004, she realized something had to change. "A good friend suggested we devise a machine to wrap the tape around the tubing."

For the next year Diana and her friend Tom worked together to create a tape-wrapping machine. Making hundreds of store-quality hoops in a day changed the BodyHoops business dramatically. Diana says, "It was exciting to see a single hoop completed in minutes. Next I wanted a hoop that did not need assembly but was easier to ship. That prompted the collapsible hoop." At first she and Tom followed the model of a tent pole that collapses with a stretchy cord inside. They didn't like the results.

Following the idea of a car windshield cover folding up, however, was successful, and their travel hoop was born. "The way the tubing was able to

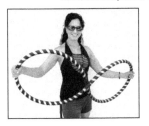

twist and coil down was almost too easy. But we still had to create a connector that would swivel to ease the circle into a figure eight and allow the hoop to fold over smartly." Folded over, the double circle is one-quarter of the hoop's full size—easy to take on a bike or on public transportation. Shortly after securing a patent, BodyHoops collaborated with Gaiam, a lifestyle company, to create the HoopBody Kit, which included a collapsible hoop and DVDs with instruction from movie star Marisa Tomei.

Light-Emitting Diode (LED)

Patrick Deluz founded the Harbin Hoop Jam (chapter 7), and invented the PsiHoops LED dance hoop. In the 1960s he had been a student at Oxford University, where he made a black-light Ping Pong game and created rooms of luminous objects in motion. Later he moved to Southern California. In 2004 hoops started showing up at the dance jams he went to. For one of the jams he hosted a '60s night with aerial performance and lighting effects synced to original music. "A friend brought vintage light-show equipment that used oil, water, and bits of colored glass. I thought a transparent hoop with lights in it would be a nice addition to the evening, but I had to figure out how to get lights inside the hoop."

Patrick couldn't find anyone with experience in lighting up hoops, so he took apart sneakers with LEDs in them to see how they were hooked up. He cut down LED pins and brooches, fit-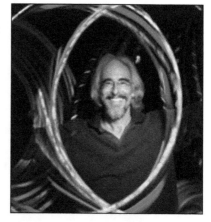ting their lights into transparent tubing. "That worked to some extent and gave me the impe-tus to build on my discoveries. Eventually I met an engineer who had used LEDs for art exhibits on the playa at Burning Man."

When Patrick was given a gift certificate that entitled him to a class with HoopGirl, he was surprised to learn that hooping classes existed. HoopGirl, Christabel Zamor, was curious about his LED hoops and invited him to meet her after class at the studio of Amy Goldstein, who had started filming *The Hooping Life*. Patrick thought, "Jeez, films about hooping—the plot thickens!"

When Christabel's group of hoopdancers was to perform at a Cirque du Soleil party celebrating the opening of the show *Ka*, she asked Patrick to make LED hoops for them to use. He says, "I filed my patent for the LED hoop and immediately took several to Las Vegas for that party. I spent the whole night running to and from my hotel room where I had set up a workbench to repair the hoops as they broke." It was a great way to pre-miere his lighted hoop and work out its bugs. Since then he has used over fifty kinds of rechargeable lights in his hoops, sometimes confounding people with too many choices.

Manufacturing involves compromise, and Patrick is continually search-ing for the ideal material. Performance characteristics of weight, flexibility, and response to heat and impact have to be considered. "One year I had a large oven and jigs made to bend custom-extruded plastic into a perfect circle. Hoopdancers loved the tougher, lighter, and clearer material."

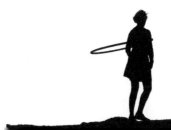

PsiHoops were large and heavy to begin with; when Patrick started making them, even professional hoopdancers were not doing many off-body moves. A forty-two-inch diameter was standard for hoopdancing. In contrast, the regulation size for rhythmic gymnastics was slightly less than thirty-six inches, and the hoop was lighter, and thinner. As a test, Patrick invited a rhythmic gymnast to use the first smaller LED hoop he made. It was faster and more maneuverable. PsiHoops became increasingly smaller and lighter, following the trend in hoopdancing. Patrick also made a sixty-inch model, roomy enough for two bodies, and a PSIchedelic instrument with a light display that is controlled by the dancer's movement. His products reflect beauty and skill, increase kinesthetic integration, and enhance visual and auditory senses.

Superhooper.org offered an LED hoop with fire spokes set into it: as the fire faded, the LEDs appeared to brighten. Try it with Quick Wicks by SynergyFireHoops.com that clamp onto any LED hoop, to ready it for fire.

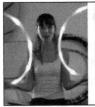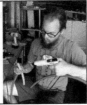

SaFire uses PsiHoops LED "twins," manipulating one with each hand.[7] V

Drew teaches us how to make the economical Polypro hoops offered at Superhooper.org. They are resizable and coil down for travel.[8] V

The Allure of Fire

Fire is a great way to light up a hoopdance if you take care, and don't mind playing with kerosene, gas, or oil.* A fire hoop has spokes around its outer edge. Each spoke has a wick at its end, which is ready to dip in fuel and set on fire. It's not just the light that attracts dancers to fire hooping. Inside a spinning fire hoop, warmth is felt swirling around the body, and the whooshing noise made by the flame is heard above all else.

Renee Kogler, founder of Cleveland Hoop Dance, says, "With a regular hoop, your hair and clothing are safe. Getting used to fire is a process. The first time I tried it my arm hair singed, but the dramatic experience of fire hooping is worth the precautions you must take."

---

* See a comparison of fuels at:
   www.templeofpoi.com/blog/2009/02/fire-and-fuel

Renee has learned to tie up or spritz long hair and wear arm coverings. Because her clothing is at risk of going up in flames, she wears fire-retardant fabric. If you play with fire, keep fuel safely contained, and never burn alone. Always have a damp blanket, a first aid kit, and a working fire extinguisher close at hand.

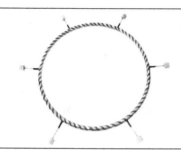

Before lighting up, check all equipment. Make sure spokes are set securely and wicks are not loose. Secure the fuel "dipping" station away from performers and audience.

Building and maintaining the tools you work with in any medium creates a more stable process and results in a more professional outcome. Juggling Inferno, a U.K. entertainment group, spins fire *poi* and staff, eats and breathes fire, and juggles with fire hoops. The group makes most of their own props and fire safety equipment; occasionally assisted by a small team of engineers they know will follow their specific requirements.

Tim Marston, founder of Juggling Inferno, got a real-world introduction to fire safety before his own career began. He was in Thailand watching a fire spinner outside of a bar. "The young man was totally lost in his own world of fire fun when a piece of flaming wick flew off the end of his staff and landed in dry brush next to the wooden bar. A few of us scrambled to find water and wet towels to put out the flames that were just getting started. The spinner kept on spinning! He was oblivious to the fact that the bar was made of wood with a thatch roof of grass and palm, which could have been burnt to the ground. The owner would have lost his business, and people could have been killed."

The incident burned a respect for the power of fire into Tim's consciousness. Instantly he saw the importance of having good quality props to work with and proper safety equipment on hand in case of fire. When his own group is asked to perform, they discuss safety with the client

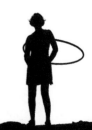

before Tim commits to a booking. "For safety," Tim says, "we never take for granted that everything will be as the client agreed, so we conduct an on-site inspection before every performance. Then we work with the client to resolve any lingering health and safety hazards." Anything, from a slippery stage to flammable décor and crowd control issues, can trip up even the most professional production. Tim also makes sure that smoke alarms

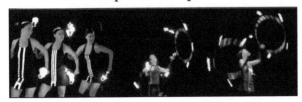

are isolated from the fire of an indoor show. "The *last* thing we want is a fire alarm going off halfway though a Juggling Inferno performance!"[9] [V]

Once you have the tools of your trade and a routine to share, Tim's e-book, *How to Sell Your Act,* has information about the business of promotion, from working with an agent to what your website will need. (See the resource section at the back of this book.)

Music That Moves You

Music brings out the movement potential in most of us, but any sound can put you in touch with your particular sense of timing: sounds of nature, the city, or silence. You can hoopdance to music in your head, beats that are naturally in your bones, or songs you may never have considered your style. Listening to classical, nostalgic, electronic, very slow melodies, or overtly popular tunes might get you out of your comfort zone and lead to untold discoveries.

Jamming

The jam band String Cheese Incident sparked the hoopdance movement. Jam Bands typically perform live music that crosses genre boundaries. They reference a diverse palette of sounds with extended improvisations that draw on blues, bluegrass, funk, jazz, rock, psychedelia, and techno. The Grateful Dead was probably the first jam band, followed by others like Phish, Dave Matthews Band, and String Cheese Incident. Groovehoops original member Michele Clark says, "I didn't realize it when I first started hooping, but listening to African music I can hear a similarity to what String Cheese Incident was playing. Their bluegrass music has references to Caribbean rhythms."

As a teenager Michele listened to early jam band music on the radio every night. "The music started out by following a structure and then built to culminate in a fever meant to induce people out of conscious thought and into their unconscious selves. It does something to your brain. I'm sure musicians feel this even more when they play in freestyle collectively. Improv dance partners experience it by moving in ways that are completely unrehearsed." Responding to the correlation between music and movement, ecstatic dancers, hoopdancers, and spinners of flow toys intuit where the music is going. Breaks in direction naturally sync with the tempo and rhythm of the music, and hooping isolations are made to pop out of and back into routines on beats.

The San Luis Obispo band Tropo is closely linked to the hoopdance community in California because its musicians understand the synergy between music and movement. Grant Leonard has been playing music with his brother Tyson and cousin Ryan Johnson for many years. As Tropo, they play electronic music with live elements of drum, guitar, keyboard, and violin. The band fluctuates the music as they *feel* what the crowd wants to hear, and they never play a song the same way twice. Grant says, "It's interactive even though some of the elements have been previously made, because Tyson can change 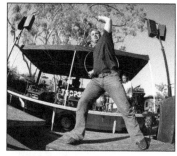 our electronic drumbeats as we improvise with our instruments." The band's early style as Rain Fur Rent had a heavy rock influence.[10] V Tropo has evolved into a synthesis of jam, techno, and house music, with breaks that reference rock and roll.[11] M

House music is mid- to up-tempo, with
   a prominent kick drum on every beat.
   The house four-on-the-floor dance beat
   is based on the technique of 1970s disco.
Techno and trance developed alongside house,
   sharing its basic beat infrastructure with
   a more synthetic sound and approach.

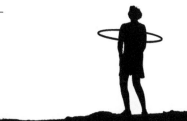

Like hoopdance, ecstatic dance is a form of interactive flow. Ecstatic dancers let their bodies respond to rhythm waves, without preconceived dance steps. Providing music for ecstatic dance is the opposite of creating popular tunes, and it is one of Grant's favorite ways to play. "We have to stretch to what is happening on the dance floor. When the crowd is large, it creates a palpable ecstatic energy."

In the San Francisco Bay Area, at some dances four to five hundred people become part of the music. They pay attention subconsciously, rather than by listening for lyrics, because their focus is on creative swaying, bumping, and dancing. Grant watches the crowd. "I see people react to what I play as if they are feeling the music as I create it. Other times I hoop on stage, taking a step back to listen and respond *without* playing." At larger venues Tropo incorporates hooping into their performance. They plan their summers around music festivals, ending with Burning Man.

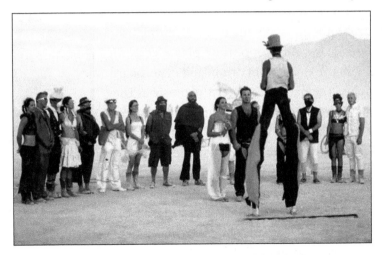

The 2009 wedding of Grant Leonard and Sharai Carpenter
at Burning Man was officiated by Kenny Gross on stilts.

Between Rain Fur Rent and Tropo, Grant saw his first hoopdancer at a High Sierra music festival. Then his housemate bought a hoop and let him use it. "I was horrible at first, but I learned to dance with that hoop. And I literally wore it out." He hooped for at least an hour every day for a year. A large window that faced him in the yard behind his house served as a mirror. Grant and Sharai moved into a 307-square-foot house with huge doors that opened up to incorporate an outside space where they could hoop without distraction, because hooping practice takes dedicated time. Grant says, "It usually takes me about forty-five minutes to get locked into the music and the rhythm of what I'm doing, but there's nothing like it for my confidence. Hoopdance taught me how to loosen up my shoulders and butt, and to flow." Sharai often spins an LED hoop while Grant plays in the band.

Working on construction projects throughout the year gives Grant financial flexibility to follow his heart. One year he made hoops for kids at a small music festival put on by a local radio station. Three years later he went back. "There were hundreds of hoops out there, and little four-year-old kids were rocking it. I can't wait to see that new wave of hoopers come up. They will take it so much further."

Mix It Up

Tisha Marina hoops with youth and teaches nonviolence in schools. She understands from experience that music affects hooping. As a child she loved to time her movements to popular music. Then a ballet class convinced her she didn't like to dance—it was too slow. She pursued track and field in high school. In college an Afro-Brazilian dance class reunited her with dance movement, and music that allowed her to embody her social and cultural expressiveness.

When she started hoopdancing, Tisha struggled to pick up moves as fast as the friend with whom she practiced. "Hoopdance was hard for me in the beginning, because my friend liked house music, with its repetitious base beat, continuous rhythm, and few words." What was Tisha missing with her friend's musical choice? Hip-hop, which allowed her to connect with her own beat.[12] [V]

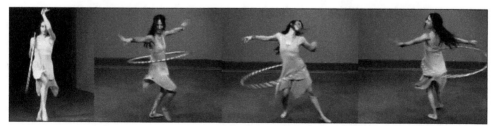

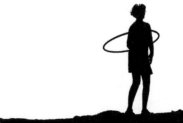

The day Tisha hoopdanced to Missy Elliott on her own, it clicked. "I realized that I had to use my kind of music with my kind of dancing."[13] [M]

Malcolm Stuart connected with dancing when he discovered his father's collection of funk music. He says, "Funk is scientifically designed to make you dance." The creative combination of notes and intervals in funk music engages the cognitive brain-body system, urging us to move. Malcolm began by listening to the great funk artists Sly and the Family Stone, William "Bootsy" Collins, and George Clinton, to name a few.[14] [M]

Caroleeena suggests that music can actually assist us in learning new moves. For instance, if you are learning the three-beat weave, three-beat music helps you to sync up the timing of your two hoops. SaFire gives an introduction to three-beat weaving.[15] [V]

Try it with one of the following songs, choosing from the genre you like best. (Samples of songs are on the book's website.) [16] [M]

"Kiss from a Rose" by Seal
"Moon River" from the *Breakfast at Tiffany's* soundtrack
"Come Away with Me" by Norah Jones
"Take It to the Limit" by the Eagles
"Natural Woman" by Aretha Franklin
"Everybody Hurts" by R.E.M.

Once you are comfortable hoopdancing to your favorite music, branch out to other genres to challenge what is natural for you. Kids often choose pop music because it is what they hear most, but when Bunny Hoop Star teaches children in Australia, she likes to surprise them by throwing in a few "curly ones"—circus tunes or some of the music she listens to at nightclubs. "I like to challenge flow with music that breaks up the usual patterns and shapes we regularly make with the hoop. I love dance music that has spirit and soul, and didgeridoo sounds that are often used in electronic music."

Christabel gave Bunny a CD of house music when they met at Burning Man in 2008. The CD is upbeat with a high 1990s vibe. When Bunny listens to it, the music brings back all the women she has hoopdanced with, "and it brings back all the singers who tell us that we can tap into our powerful female energy and have fun being super hot, playful, and successful. Madonna, Blondie, and the Pussycat Dolls make me feel like I can do anything."[17] [M]

Bunny also likes the tribal beats of the Beats Antique. They accompanied Miss Rosie's belly dance and hoopdance performance at Burning Man in 2009.[18] [V]

Drumming for Hooping

When he fell in love with Julia Hartsell, drumming led Scott Crews to an interest in hooping. "Julia hired me to play at a swank wedding gig; we fell in love through the course of it and into the evening." Scott became a drummer at the age of thirteen, starting with the kit his grandfather, Marvin Crews, handed down to him. Drumming had been Marvin's hobby, but Scott never heard him play. He discovered the kit in Marvin's basement and played it there occasionally until it was given to him outright.

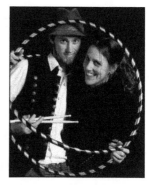

The cyclical nature of drum beats fused Scott's music with Julia's hooping. Their flow intertwined so naturally that even when they practice in different rooms, their mistakes can affect one another. Scott says, "You would expect it to affect *her* concentration when I miss a beat, but the interesting thing is that sometimes *my* beat falters when she botches a move, even if I can't see her."

When Scott plays music with his friend Osker, it consists of live drumming with remixes and on-the-spot resequencing of recorded loops. It is meditative, repetitive, and cyclical. It breathes, flows, and works well with hoopdancing. Scott likes to shoulder hoop, knows some tricks, and once got into a hoop flow listening to music at a festival, but he says, "Mostly I'm not good enough to hoop as rhythmically as I'd like. However, I'm very thankful that hooping has become a dance form, as I've always played my drums for dancers."[19] [V]

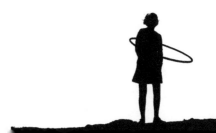

The Playlist

To add consistency or variety to hooping practice, songs can be arranged in a specific order or shuffled in a music player. Adam Parson, a visual artist in Indiana, learned to hoop on a visit to Berkeley and has sent me several playlists since. "It Doesn't Have to Be English" includes songs I automatically want to hoop to, especially these three:[20] M

> "Only You" by Praise from the album of the same name
> "Wombo Lombo" by Angélique Kidjo from *Fifa*
> "Martha's Song" by Deep Forest from *Boheme.*

Laura Marie compiles a monthly playlist for the Internet friends and followers of Hooping Harmony. Her selections constantly vary in style, from hip-hop and world music to tunes from the 1940s and 1960s or the quieter side of hooping. Her sacred mix includes:[21] M

> The Goddess Alchemy Project for rap
> Ash Dargan for didgeridoo
> David Starfire for tribal sutras.

SaFire encourages us to hoop through the evolution of popular dance by compiling sound bites from historically influential songs. The idea is to hoopdance in the style that the era evokes in you. A playlist for hooping through the history of music could go like this:[22] M

> "London in the Rain" by Variety Lab, 2001
> "Macarena" by Los del Río, 1995
> "Thriller" by Michael Jackson, 1980
> "Rocket Man" by Elton John, 1972
> "I Fall to Pieces" by Patsy Cline, 1961
> "Blue Suede Shoes" by Elvis, 1955
> "Rum and Coca-Cola" by the Andrews Sisters, 1945
> and so forth, back as far as you want to go.

DJ Spin Sisters

Hoopdancing and sustained spinning are frequently practiced at events where electronic music is played by DJs who sample previously recorded music. Sophia Mavrides is an ecstatic dancing DJ who is known for leaving her turntables to join dancers on the floor. "I weave sounds to create a unified field of consciousness with music that includes funk, Latin, Brazilian, Balkan beats, trance, and euro lounge. Whatever gets people moving." And she hoops.

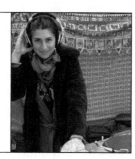

Sophia makes "mixes" that are similar to playlists. They are compilations of songs that follow each other to tell a story or systematically increase energy in various parts of the body as you listen or dance.

At the Harbin Hoop Jam Sophia gave me an introduction to the simple technique she uses for "spinning sound." She listens through headphones to CDs on two players, amplifying tracks on one and lowering the volume of the other near the end of songs, or at a break in the music, when the beats make a good match. Her process is influenced by mood, and it begins with time spent finding the music she samples. "I mix new tunes in with ones I have used before because the better I know the beats, the more my heart will be in what I play. If I know the artists personally, all the better; I can feel and transmit their intention when I play their music." The DJ is a channel for mixing energy as well as music. Through technique and intuition Sophia's choices are like a call and response. Her rhythm affects dancers on the floor. Their reaction in turn informs what she chooses to play next. In the process, she strives for a balance between being receptive and stepping in to make decisions. "Like steering a ship," she admits, "once you get off course, it's hard to bring it back. If a DJ sits back too much, the music will become overly random."

Some DJs stay within the headset, looking out but never joining the dancers. When Sophia wants to go onto the dance floor during a session, she programs a series of songs in advance. "The difference between listening through headphones and feeling it from within the crowd, out in

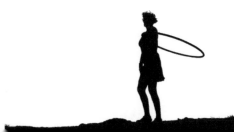

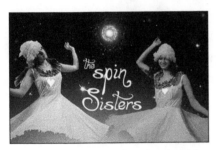

front, is significant. The perception of energy and the actual experience of that energy can be completely different. DJ-ing is like dancing, and your partner is the room." Sophia and her partner, Kat Giacona, are known as the Spin Sisters. While working individually, they each began to twirl during spells they took on the dance floor. Together they decided to wear skirts and to twirl more often as an ecstatic moving meditation.[23] V

Sophia says, "Sustained turning to music puts you right in your center; if you are off center at all, you can't do it. DJ-ing together is twice as hard, requiring more surrender, but Kat and I have found a rhythm that works." Sophia's work is informed by Gabrielle Roth's five energies: flowing, staccato, chaos, lyrical, and stillness. "As I look out at the dancers on the floor, thinking in terms of the different parts of our energetic selves helps me to see when a change in tone is required." Her beats are more rhythmic for hoopdancers, because consistent patterns that are sustained overlong will induce boredom for them. She raises and lowers the musical vibration, balancing "dark and bassy" with "lyrical heart" to take rhythm to "completion with cohesion." She'll see you on the dance floor!

Create a Costume without Sewing

Materials: fitted, cast-off T-shirt, sharp scissors,
ruler, pen, circle pattern, straight pins.

Peepholes:

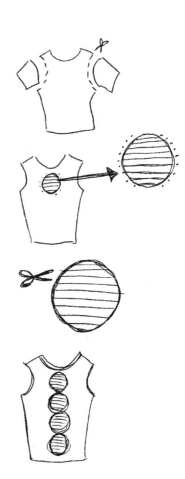

Step 1: Pick a T-shirt that fits snugly.
Cut off the sleeves, and put them aside
for the armband project. Place the shirt
on a flat surface inside out.

Step 2: Cut a circle pattern from a grocery
bag or heavy paper. Draw lines across it at
quarter- or half-inch intervals.

Step 3: Place the pattern on the shirt, making
a small mark on each side of every pattern
line. Connect the dots into lines on the shirt.

Step 4: Cut along each line, then gently
stretch the shirt from side to side
until the fabric starts to roll. You
have created a peephole!

Try creating shapes with several circles,
alternating the direction of the lines,
or overlapping the circles.
Anything goes.

Armbands:

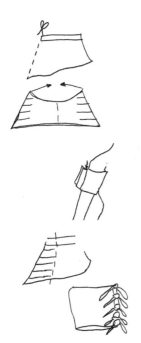

Step 1: Cut along the fold opposite the sleeve's seam, and open. The seam is in the middle.

Step 2: Wrap the fabric around your upper arm, pinching it snugly, and pin together.

Step 3: Remove the fabric without dislodging the pins. Mark at one-inch intervals along the cut edge, then cut through the double thickness from the edge, to the pin line.

Step 4: Remove the pins, and tie the right and left strips together in knots. It's ready to wear.

Pattern by Annieland.

Chapter Nine Links

www.HoopDanceBook.com/chapter9

1. *Chest and Shoulder Hooping Tutorial.* Feb. 9, 2009.

2. *Shakti Sunfire Performs with Airaligned—Hoop Dance.* Oct. 30, 2009.

3. *Alexis of the Funkshine Hoop Troop in Tampa, FL.* Dec. 25, 2009.

4. *Seattle Fashion Week 2011 Act 3 Hoop Dance.* May 11, 2011.

5. *Makeup by GlitterGirl.* Jul. 30, 2009.

6. *Explaining the Maghoop Trio Set.* Jul. 27, 2011.

7. *SaFire's New Hoops! psihoops.com.* Nov. 19, 2009.

8. *Episode 1—Prepping Clear Tubing.* Feb. 15, 2012.

9. *Juggling Inferno Fire Shows.* Oct. 13, 2011.

10. *Rain Fur Rent—"Compared to What."* Feb. 15, 2010.

11. "Interweave" by Tropo. 2011.

12. *Tisha Marina, Hoop Dance.* Sep. 26, 2011.

13. "Play That Beat" by Missy Elliott. 2003.

14. Malcolm's Funk Music:

    "Everyday People" by Sly and the Family Stone. 1968.

    "Stretchin' Out (In a Rubber Band)" by Bootsy Collins. 1976.

    "Loopzilla" by George Clinton. 1982.

15. *Hooping Tutorial: Introduction to 3 Beat Weave with Mini Hoops.* Nov. 26, 2009.

16. Three-Beat Music:

    "Kiss from a Rose" by Seal. 1994.

    "Moon River" by Henry Mancini. 1961.

    "Come Away with Me" by Norah Jones. 2003.

    "Take It to the Limit" by The Eagles. 1975.

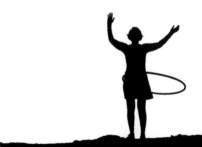

"(You Make Me Feel Like) Natural Woman" by Aretha Franklin. 1967.

"Everybody Hurts" by R.E.M. 1992.

17. "Material Girl" by Madonna. 2002.

"The Tide Is High" by Blondie. 1967.

"Don't Cha" by The Pussycat Dolls. 2005.

18. *Miss Rosie with Beats Antique Burning Man 2009.* Sep. 10, 2009.

19. *University Mall Performance.* Nov. 3, 2008.

20. It Doesn't Have to Be English:

"Only You" by Praise. 1991.

"Wombo Lombo" by Angélique Kidjo. 1995.

"Martha's Song" by Deep Forest. 1995.

21. Hooping Harmony Sacred Mix:

"Secrets" by The Goddess Alchemy Project. 2008.

"Sunrise Song" by Ash Dargan. 2002.

"Mystic Whomp" by David Starfire. 2010.

22. History-of-music Playlist:

"London in the Rain" by Variety Lab. 2001.

"Macarena" by Los del Río. 1995.

"Thriller" by Michael Jackson. 1980.

"Rocket Man" by Elton John. 1972.

"I Fall to Pieces" by Patsy Cline. 1961.

"Blue Suede Shoes" by Elvis. 1955.

"Rum and Coca-Cola" by the Andrews Sisters. 1945

23. *DJ SpinSisters at The Groove Garden Beltane Bump May 2010.* Jun. 13, 2010.

TEN

Related Flow Arts

The line is a dot that went for a walk.
—Paul Klee, visual artist

Flow is a state of mind that can be achieved through a variety of movement disciplines. Hoopdancers borrow technique from traditional dance, juggling, yoga, and martial arts. Likewise, dancers, yogis, martial artists, and object manipulators incorporate hoops and hoopdance technique into their practice.

Dance

On solid ground, belly dance teaches Adelaide Marcus to flow from side to side. Her movements tell a story of passion, spirituality, and dreams. In the air she balances along a communal midline, as she and Sam Salwei create an acrobatic fusion. When she moves even a hand, her fingers follow each other like waves rolling through water.

Adelaide and her sister Leilainia (The Shimmy Sisters) grew up belly dancing with their mother, an art handed down from the Syrian side of their family. Adelaide incorporates hooping into both belly dance and her daring forms of contorted

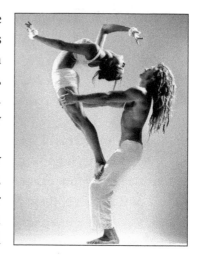

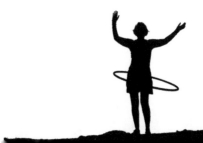

balancing. "It takes a super-awareness of contradictory movement disciplines in order to balance solidly while moving gracefully." As a belly dancer first, she hoopdances with extremely fluid body lines.[1] [V]

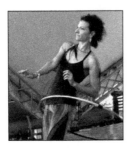

Modern dance combines extremes of graceful and angular choreography to tell a story. When the extreme you want is to slow the hoop down, Anah Reichenbach suggests rolling it around your core. The ability to use your abdominal muscles like a belly dancer is helpful. In a group, you can borrow technique from tribal belly dancers to communicate cues to each other for transitions through body language. In Pacific Island hula dance, mime-like gestures traditionally accompany songs to illustrate oral history. Anah modifies "hula hands" from this form of dance to help beginning hoopdancers get used to reaching in all directions. It's a variation on hula "vamp arms" and "the sun." (See instructions at the end of the chapter.)

Ecstatic dance gives us a model for contemplative movement, as a meditation on music that shifts brain patterns from cognitive (beta) to more

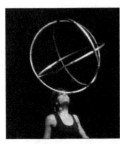

insightful (alpha) waves. Michele Clarke discovered ecstatic dance on her way to finding the hoop. American Indian hoop dancers use multiple hoops to make shapes that represent elements of ritual ceremony or sacred stories. Hoopdancers like Michele flow their hoops into similar configurations, such a globe that can be made with two or more hoops interlaced with one another.

Rich Porter and Spiral broke down components of dance theory for their program Hoop Technique. They created a structure for understanding and applying four essential concepts. Whether you choreograph or improvise, awareness of these elements can make your hoopdance more dynamic.

- Space: the relationship of body and hoop to surroundings. Are you interacting with your environment?

- Energy: conscious application of physical and emotional movement. Does your movement reflect your intention?

- Time: speed, acceleration, direction changes, tempo, and beat. Can you vary action for surprises that will make your dance more engaging?

- Flow: effortless transition guided by inspiration, challenge, and expertise. Can you let go of discursive thoughts to be moved by muscle memory?

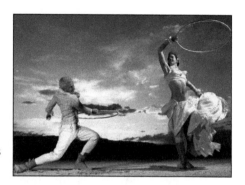

Choreography versus Improvisation

In flow, each movement builds upon the previous one to inform the next, whether with preconceived intention or spontaneous impulse. For instance, I might choreograph a routine in which I memorize, in my body through repeated practice, a series of moves such as core hooping, to lasso above the head, to weaving with jump-through, and back to waist hooping. If I practice these to music, eventually the beats of the song recall the intended moves without me thinking rationally about them. Or I could listen to any song and let the beats evoke spontaneous movement. Either method requires drawing on the spatial awareness, timing, and energy I have embodied, beyond learning intellectually, through my hoop practice.

Artists at the Canopy Studio Repertory Company in Athens, Georgia, use hooping routines combined with aerial dance to tell dramatic stories through nuanced action. Choreographer Dana Skelton says, "By choosing how we use our efforts, we learn a process for turning ordinary moves into flowing dramatic dance." The way movement is conceived and executed is all-important. If a routine calls for moving the hoop from the side to the front of the body, the hoopdancer's physical intention within the dramatic situation conveys the meaning of that shift.

For instance, you can grab a hoop tightly and thrust it into space, or hold it with a slightly open palm and guide it to the same place. A thrust and a glide each deliver a different message. When the dancer is in flow, the message comes from a place of deep physical understanding. In

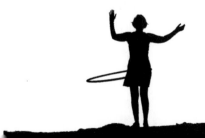

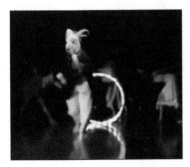

Canopy Studio performances, a pirate-theme show might use hoops as sirens of the sea, swooping and beckoning against billowing blue fabric. For *Alice in Wonderland* they evoke a fall through time, with dancers turning LED hoops into a lighted black hole, revealing the White Rabbit. Dana says, "When people see trapeze and other aerial dance in our shows, they may be intimidated to try it, but everyone can pick up a hoop and give it a spin."

The paradox of flow is that creating the space for profound release requires disciplined effort in order to relinquish the thinking mind to the movement. In a choreographed production, practice readies the dancer to be totally involved with intention and to flow. Even so, Baxter sees choreography as a restriction in the improvisational style he developed for the HoopPath program. His route toward flow does not have a preconceived notion of what the next move will look like, but rather calls for unleashing what you feel immediately moved to do. This method relies on "a sweet surrender" to the "providential grace" of each person's self-development. "It's really tough to hit all of your marks when you have a swimming hoop moving around you. If you don't hit the 'ta-da' in a choreographed piece, it looks sloppy. With improv, if you hit, you hit, but that's not the goal." However, if what the dancer is moved to do next is a perfect expression of his or her feelings, it often *looks* choreographed to an audience.

How will you arrive at this perfect expression of your internal sense of "ta-da"? Through practice for personal regeneration, with no single movement taking precedence. When flow emerges from this type of direction, physical expression is revealed in spontaneous action. Baxter's students learn to respond to what is happening inside themselves rather than to strive to be like their teacher. He calls this an "emerge or die" process.[2] Ⓥ

Flow Toys

Props, such as a hoop in hoopdance, or a ball in contact juggling, are sometimes called "toys," because they facilitate creative playfulness. Play leads to inventiveness, flexibility, and resilience, qualities that help flow artists create movement that has beauty, the power to move us emotionally. Following is a list of the most common flow toys.

Ball (for contact juggling): A ball is held while it is moved and rolled over the body, so that it appears to be suspended in space or to float on its own.

Club: A traditional prop used by jugglers, the club's center of balance is near its wide body below a slim handle. When an object manipulator uses two or more clubs, juggling becomes secondary to the paths and shapes made with them in space.

Fire Fan: Modeled on flamenco fans, fire fans, with four or five wicks on each fan, are used in pairs. They are spun with a series of finger grips.

Hoop: This tubular circle of any size can be spun around the body or manipulated by hand while dancing, with or without fire.

Poi: Pairs of cord or chain with balls or wicks attached are swung around the body. Knowledge of *poi* can help in learning to spin other props.

Staff: The martial arts staff is a long, thick, stick-shaped object that can be used as a weapon. It is manipulated for dramatic effect, with or without fire.

Wand: Originally used for magic shows, the wand has been redesigned specifically for object manipulation and is sometimes called a "stick."

Proficiency gained through repetition and insight leads to letting go, the giving up of conscious control, which is necessary for flow in both meditation and performance. Using a prop does not automatically induce flow; getting there takes practice. Tim Marston, founder of the fire-performance group Juggling Inferno, works on prop control and footwork for hours upon hours, alone and without fire, in order to flow on stage with his group.[3] V

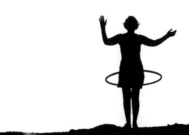

With each manipulation of a prop, the successful artist delivers an emotional message, be it provocation with an isopop (the hoop popping out of a seemingly stationary hoop revolution) or fear, with a great many clubs threatening to foil a performer with impossibility.

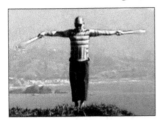

Khan Wong produces the annual Flow Show in San Francisco to present professional and developing flow artists. He was mesmerized by fire dancers the first time he saw them spinning *poi* at Burning Man. A desire to join them inspired him to take classes in *poi.* Then he began working with clubs.[4] V

Deciding to add a third prop to his repertoire, Khan tried hooping, and it quickly took over his practice. He says, "The hoop seems to be the most accessible of flow toys and the one that has the greatest range."

Laurie Hobbs concurs: "Even though my spiraling vortex motions *feel* terrific with *poi,* they often *look* much better with the hoop. I think I was trying to hoop from the start—even with *poi*—I just hadn't found my tool yet. As soon as I got a hoop in my hand, everything clicked."

The Ball and Small Hoops

Michael Moschen pioneered hoop isolations by perfecting what he referred to as "dynamic manipulation," a method of ball juggling also known as "contact juggling" and often simply referred to as "object manip-

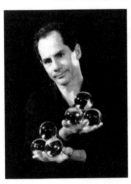

ulation." He grew up in Greenfield, Massachusetts, where he began to juggle at the age of twelve with his friend and neighbor Penn Jillette. Jillette later became half of the magic duo Penn & Teller. Moschen went on tour with clown Bob Berky as the Alchemedians, and then gravitated toward performance art. In 1990 he received a five-year MacArthur Genius Grant to pursue his research into the dynamic properties of objects in space and time. He developed precision hand movements, with body rolls, stalls, and isolations, that make a ball appear to have its own life force.

European artist Adrien Mondot combines techniques for object manipulation, like Moschen's, with dance and digital projection. In his video trailer for *Cinematique,* letters of the alphabet flow from his flashlight, illuminating dark space. As his methodical movements accelerate, he swirls virtual ABCs in circles and loops, and performers dance frantically on a disappearing grid.[5] [V]

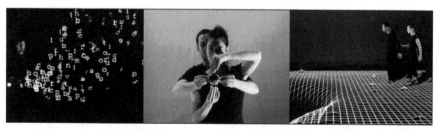

Translated to the hoop, dynamic manipulation is called "contact hooping." It incorporates ball technique with neo-vaudevillian hoop rolling, a sleight-of-hand technique that makes a hoop seem to animate itself. In Oakland, California, Matt "Poki" McCorkle and Brian Thompson perform contact hooping as Code Red: Circus Conspiracy. They synchronize hoop sequencing and patterning with precision and illusion.[6] [V]

Patterns in Play

Rainbow Michael, of Synergy Fire Hoops, uses geometry to inform and describe his practice of manipulating props, which include small hoops. His long-exposure photos of *poi* with LED lights reveal flower shapes and

other sacred geometric symbols, like the pentacle or six-pointed star, that have been used in pagan and other religious cosmologies for thousands of years. "The audience may be aware of the meaning in shapes created with flow toys," he explains, "or they may simply take in the breathtaking electricity that is generated by them. Either way, the universal language of pattern is accessible to all." His strength and agility 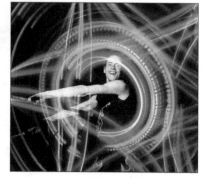 are reinforced by years of yoga practice. His hooping is graceful, and his props seem to float, glide, and fly with dynamic momentum.[7] [V]

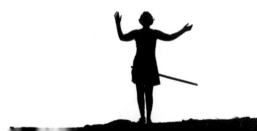

Cross-Pollination

Traditional circus artists were secretive about the illusions they created; they rarely disclosed information about how tricks were executed. In contrast, festivals like Burning Man, and sharing over the Internet, foster an open-source model in the flow arts community. When spinners come up with new material, they not only share it with friends in person but also post a how-to video on the Web. People all over the world build upon it and post further refinements.

Hoopdancing is energized by the practice of spinning, which it shares with other props, but the hoop has an advantage. You can translate off-body movement to hooping, but you can also get inside a hoop. That doesn't translate back to off-body-only flow toys. Nadia Sophia, a hooping fire performer with martial arts training, says, "Everything that you learn with *poi* you can do with other props, but sometimes the moves look better with a hoop. For instance, slowing down while hooping can look awesome, whereas with *poi* it might look sloppy." Circus Conspiracy compares and contrasts *poi* and hoops.[8] V

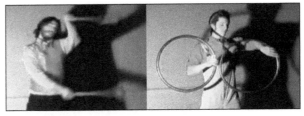

Fire fans are so elegant that you don't have to do much of anything to make them look good. That gives them an edge. They are also difficult to manipulate in complex ways. Grimm of Incendium Arts demonstrates crossover technique from fans to hoops.[9] V

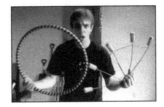

At the largest scale, a prop called the simple wheel has been used extensively in Chinese and French circuses. At Hoopcamp 2010 participants

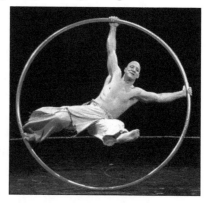

who experienced the wheel were emboldened to move in increasingly dramatic ways when wielding their smaller hoops around themselves. The incarnation of the wheel they used was developed in the early 2000s by Daniel Cyr, and has become known as the Roue Cyr, or Cyr Wheel. It is a metal hoop generally made to match the manipulator's height plus his or her fist, which adds two to three inches. For example, a six-foot-diameter wheel would be used by a performer approximately five feet, eight inches tall. The wheel is manipulated both off-body and as a vehicle with feet as well as hands grasping its inner edge.[10] V

Yoga

As toddlers we learn to move through trial and error, developing unconscious competence. Beyond the playpen we take instruction, but we don't always know the underlying principles of what we are taught. For instance, exercise instructors often call for "chest out, shoulders back, and chin in." How often is it explained that we are to engage the hyoid muscles that surround the u-shaped bone in the neck as we lift and expand the chest while keeping it flexible? Other common instructions such as "find your sit bones" and "move from your center" require engaging the psoas muscles (pronounced "SO-az") located deep in the abdomen. They are a key component in developing fluid self-carriage. While the psoas muscles perform in conjunction with surface muscles, they are the only ones that directly connect the spine to the legs and are often a missing link in hoopdance.

In yoga as in hoopdance, muscles, bones, organs, and breath shift in relationship to each other. Yoga helps us to accomplish flow in hoopdance

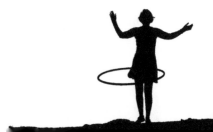

by training the body to mindfully lift, lengthen, and flex specific muscles in order to move into and hold the various *asana* (pronounced "AHsahnah"), postural shapes made by the body with support from the breath. Once a shape is achieved, breath is used to lengthen muscles, and to let go of tension around particular bones as we relax more deeply into a pose or flow seamlessly into the next position. Imagine or try the following partial sun salutation.

Inhale while raising your arms overhead, lengthening the spine and lifting the rib cage with the palms of your hands facing each other. As you exhale, fold your upper body forward from the hips, keeping the spine long and not rounding your back, and then drop your hands toward your feet. Legs can be straight without locking the knees or flexed to prevent strain. Relax your head and shoulders toward the floor. As you inhale in this folded position, breathe into your back body, and feel it expand. As you exhale, relax more deeply into the pose, as if your sit bones are rising as your head sinks toward the floor.

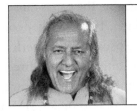

Laughter is a wonderful breathing tool. Like the yoga "breath of fire," laughter pumps air out from the lungs rhythmically. Laugh while contracting your abdominal muscles, keeping your chest and shoulders open. Then pump out a continuous "ha ha ha" to the rhythm of clapping your hands. Now try it while hooping, as you turn opposite to the direction of your hoop. You get a powerful burst of energy.

> Ramesh Pandey (Yogi Ramesh), known as the laughing yogi, tells us that when we laugh silently, our lungs, heart, kidneys, and other organs dance.[11] [V]

Muscle Memory

Hoopdance instructor and social worker Kaye Anderson alternates Ashtanga yoga with hoop practice. Together these disciplines give her constantly renewed perspective on areas of her training where she has progressed and those that need more attention. Ashtanga yoga relies on specific postures done in exact sequence. As the body learns the poses through repetition, muscle memory is gained. Over time, the mind is relieved of striving for an appropriate shape, allowing the intelligence of the body to take over.

There are six series of Ashtanga poses, and many students, including Kaye, spend years learning the first sequence. "I'm a fidgeter," Kaye says. "I have a hard time sitting still and get distracted by my thoughts. Hooping helps me find my meditative spot, the place of mindfulness others get to in yoga. I get there by spinning around in circles, which supports my yoga practice." With her yoga teacher, Melanie Green, Kaye offers "Hooping and Yoga" workshops. Not to be confused with AcroYoga hooping, these classes use each discipline alternately rather then combining them. After warming up, Melanie guides a series of yoga exercises that call upon resistance and yielding, such as stretching the side and back body, to achieve various poses. Kaye then shows us an equivalent series of hoopdance moves that require elongation in the side and back body to achieve dance moves with the hoop. It's an hour and a half of breath-supported, energizing fun.

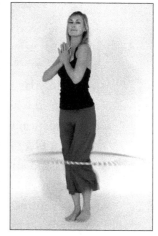

Contact Yoga

Yoga brings us into a state of flow through a surrender to trust in all that we are. This principle is heightened when we practice with another person. Remember playing "airplane" as a kid or as a parent "flying" kids on your feet? The adult's feet extend upward. The exhilarated child balances with arms outstretched, flying. That experience of playful, fearless freedom within a secure and proficient relationship is the essence of contact yoga, which flows from a long tradition of partner yoga, first documented by yoga master Tirumalai Krishnamacharya in 1938. Krishnamacharya died at the age of one hundred in 1989, passing his teachings on to B. K. S. Iyegar and others who have also become influential teachers.

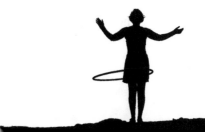

Contact yoga has been practiced in California at Santa Monica's Muscle Beach since the 1990s, and the term "AcroYoga" was coined to describe it when Jenny Sauer-Klein and Jason Nemer wrote the original *AcroYoga Flight Manual* in 2000.[12]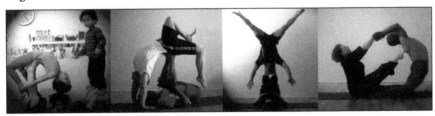

Pairing partners for contact, "base" yogis remain solidly connected to the ground while "flyers" are completely aerial, grounded only by points of connection with the base—such as hands, hips, feet, knees, backs, and so forth. Flyers are often lighter and bases stronger, but reverse or equal weights and strength can also work well if there is sufficient skill. Group contact yoga is similar to adagio, the more advanced multipartner balancing routines that originated in the Eastern European circus. Contact yoga, whether with partners or in groups, requires trust, communication, and playfulness. With dedicated practice, bases develop an innate sense of balance, flyers gain serious core strengthening, and both become more flexible. The outcome is fun, promotes fitness, and leads to meditative states of flow.

Daring to Fly

Claire French (Frenchy) founded Frenchy Productions in New Zealand. She attributes her success as a contact yoga flyer in part to the hoop. "Picking up the hoop has allowed me to play. I never had that as a fat kid who had difficulties at home."

As an adult Frenchy had weighed as much as 340 pounds, and before she could start hooping, she had to lose weight. She began by reeducating herself about eating habits and portion sizes and then added loads of exercise that included yoga, snowboarding, and bicycling. "It takes a complete change in lifestyle to lose half of your body weight and keep it off. Diets don't work by themselves. For me the key was finding exercise that I love so that I kept on doing it." When she took dance and movement courses at the Liverpool Institute of Performing Arts, it was difficult for her to keep up with slimmer classmates. In modern dance class she was often given "the man's role," when lifting a partner up was called for.

After Frenchy completed her college degree in community arts she trained young people in production skills at a Manchester radio station. She continued to hoop-dance and kept an eye on her weight, but when she tried contact yoga at the U.K. Hoop Gathering and at classes in Manchester, she couldn't fly. She couldn't imagine how light she actually had become, or even that it was physically possible for someone to lift her. "I had a block about being heavy, which I was unable to shift out of my psyche. Even though it mattered less and less that

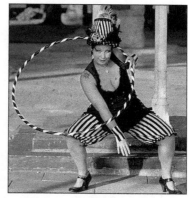

I was once massively overweight, part of me held onto that old self-image." Then she had a breakthrough experience in 2010.

At the Harbin Hoop Jam in California, Frenchy played with graceful abandon. She had not worried about her weight for a long time, and she decided to try partner yoga once again. In a group exercise, each person took a turn at being base, flyer, and spotter (the person watching out for the safety of the other two). When it was Frenchy's turn to fly, she had a hard time. "I was so uncomfortable with the idea of someone lifting me up that I battled against relaxing and letting go completely." The caring friendliness of the people in the group, together with the supportive nature of the setting, allowed her to share and shed her mental block. "Everyone was rooting for me to do it. I felt the whole group helping me and after a couple of tries—Yes! I let go for the first time in my life, and I felt light and rather weightless."

If anyone had told Frenchy years before that she would make her living by swinging a plastic circle around her waist in front of thousands of people, she would have said, "You are mad!" Now she travels the world with her hoop, performing with fire, and getting her childhood back. She exclaims, "I get younger every year." [13] [V]

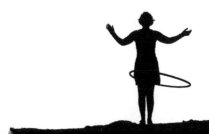

Extreme Fusion

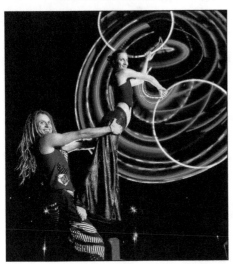

Yoga provides Sam Salwei with a window into the root of all movement, whether he is experimenting with other forms of physical activity on his own or performing partner yoga, balancing, and hooping with Adelaide Marcus.

Sam met Adelaide at an advanced YogaSlackers AcroYoga training. Combining his acrobatics teaching technique and her performance skills, they cotaught "Discovering Harmony in Duality" for acrobatics, hoopdance, and belly dance on the slackline. I was intimidated by the line when Sam introduced me to it at the Harbin Hoop Jam, but his gentle reassurance and steady guidance soon put me at ease.

A slackline is a ribbon of nylon webbing anchored between two points as an undulating ground on which to walk, play, and, in Sam's case, perform yoga poses. Like a trampoline, the slackline moves up and down. It also moves left and right. Whereas a tightrope walker uses a pole to balance on a taut and thin wire suspended at a great height, the slackline is an inch or two wide, close to the ground, and controlled by the body alone. Balancing on the slackline requires continual redistribution of weight in micro-movements.

As a teenager Sam's ideas about movement began to change. He fell in love with nature and the art of survival when his family moved to North Dakota. The following year he learned to drive. "After a ten-thousand-mile road trip and countless hours of driving dirt and muddy roads, the vehicle became an extension of my body. As I look back, I realize that I was no longer comfortable with the free-form activities of my early childhood, like swimming idly in a pool. Instead I began to seek out ways to contain and challenge my movements." He immersed himself in the art of rock climbing, in which yoga helped him to be just as strong when pulling or pushing himself up a structure. Then he met Sean O'Conner while visiting friends in North Dakota and hitched a ride east with him. At a rest stop Sean set up a slackline, and Sam loved its simplicity. In less than a minute he was hooked. "I could not stand on it for more than two seconds, but every time I tried, I felt a little closer to gaining the balance." On the road again, Sam heard about his new friend's idea for a book titled *Yoga for Slackers*. He took the words to heart and later formed a YogaSlackers team. The team performs extreme sports all over the world.

Initially it took Sam three months to successfully walk across a one-inch wide, thirty-five-foot-long nylon line. Then he headed to New Zealand to study outdoor recreation and brought a line with him. Traveling around between his coursework, he taught slacklining to other travelers. Back in the United States he teamed up with Jason Magness. They released a Slackasana DVD, and developed the eLine to facilitate flow play and yoga practice, moving over sixty asana and a few ten- to fifteen-minute vinyasa flows onto the line. The eLine's tension can be varied quickly and easily— slack for freestyle movement, slightly slack for yoga practice, or tight for performing acrobatic tricks.[14] V

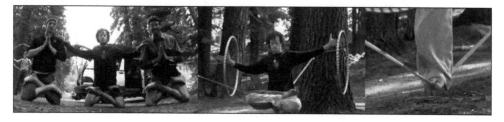

Martial Arts

The martial arts teach us that a small force can build momentum large enough to overcome an opponent in combat. This concept translates to the practice of hoopdance as the velocity of your hoop and the gestures of your body create momentum through action and reaction. Nadia Sophia uses martial arts to communicate with and discipline herself rather than as self-defense, even though many of the types she has practiced are based on combat. After she earned a black belt in tae kwon do, she set out to find the perfect dojo, teacher, and group of people with whom to train.

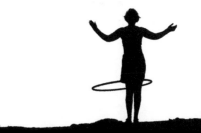

She tried ninjutsu, aikido, Muay Thai kickboxing, and Brazilian jiujitsu. None lasted very long. But with capoeira Nadia finally found her martial art "family" in Memphis.

Tae kwon do employs a system of blocks, kicks, punches, and open-handed strikes, using the reach and strength of the legs to maximize power.

Ninjutsu Survivalist Technique utilizes personal power as well as hand weapons to perform extraordinary actions.

Aikido redirects an attacker's momentum with centering and turning movements, requiring very little physical strength.

Muay Thai kickboxing features punches, kicks, standing grappling, and head butts to wear down or knock out an opponent.

Brazilian jiujitsu focuses on grappling and ground fighting to allow smaller opponents to successfully defend against opponents with superior reach.

Capoeira employs contact improvisation acted out by two or more persons within a circle to develop strength and agility.

Capoeira for Hoopdancers

Capoeira movement is something like break dancing, beautifully fluid and

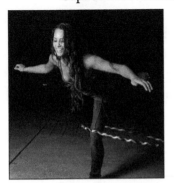

acrobatic. Some styles emphasize fighting, but Nadia loves it as a communal activity. "You get together to move, play musical instruments, and sing. I'm not good at singing, but you don't have to be good at it for capoeira."

Originally developed by African slaves as early as the sixteenth century, capoeira's music and dance was used as a cover while training for revolt in Brazil. Music creates a sacred space within and around the circle called a *roda* (pronounced "hoda"). At least one *berimbau* is required for musical accompaniment, which controls the *roda*. The *berimbau* looks like a four-foot bow and arrow with one string along its curved neck and a gourd at the bottom for amplification. Earlier forms of the berimbau were used in Africa and the diaspora during rituals for speaking with ancestors. The simple instrument was easily made of discarded wood, gourds, and wire to generate the musical style that developed along with capoeira.[15] [M]

In capoeira, if the music is low and quiet, the game becomes slow and fluid, dancers bending low to the ground. Up-tempo music prompts clapping and energetic dancing, with flips and bold stances. When capoeira was used to ready participants for combat, changes in the music told fighters inside the circle when the enemy was nearby. If authorities that might shut them down were present, the music calmed, and movements became seemingly innocent.

As a game, capoeira can be played for hours on end with repetitive call and response melodies following one after the other, sung in Brazilian Portuguese, and setting the style and energy of the *roda*. All the songs have the same four-quarter signature rhythm. Once a few of these songs are heard, they can be easily learned on the spot while playing within the circle.

In Nadia's capoeira class there was an average of eight men, and she was generally the only woman. Everyone agreed that capoeira works better with a female presence dancing in the circle, so her teammates were glad she was there. When Nadia hoopdances to contemporary music, she recalls capoeira's graceful bending, kicking, and swiveling.[16] [V]

Hoopoeira

Zach Fischer and Marria Grace, of the Vegetable Circus and Boston Hoop Troop, are a fusion team. Together they are super ninja hoopers. Using Marria's hoopdance technique and Zach's martial-arts training, they teach Ninja Hoops classes as well as park core for adults and children. Zach says, "Capoeira is geared toward improvisational movement, going with the flow, and working with what's around you. Hoopoeira evolved when I was learning to hoop. If I didn't know what move to make next, I dropped into a capoeira position." Zach and Marria are playful hoopdancers.[17] [V]

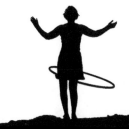

Anah's Hula Hands Exercise

Hooping on the waist, keep shoulders, rib cage, and hips facing forward, and your hoop level on the horizontal plane throughout.

- Reach both arms and hands over to one side. Raise them overhead, lifting the rib cage. Lower arms and hands gracefully to the other side.

- Sweep the arms and hands out in front, on their way back to the first side.

- Now put these movements together to make graceful, sweeping circles while continuing to keep the hoop on an even keel.

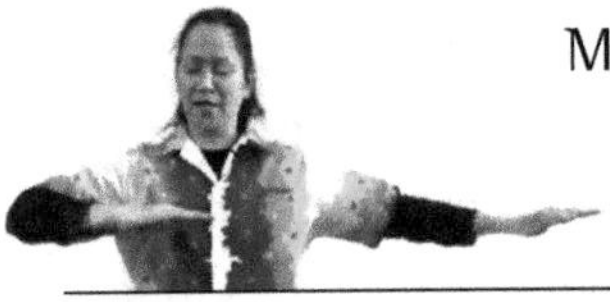

Makalina Gallagher teaches the movement of arms and hands in Pacific Island hula dancing.[18] [V]

Chapter Ten Links

www.HoopDanceBook.com/chapter10

1. *Art By Adelaide Presents- Gypsy Hoop Fusion at the San Diego Burning Man Film Festival.* Apr. 10, 2011.

2. *Hoop Practice Principles: Baxter on "Emerge or Die."* Nov. 30, 2010.

3. *Singles, doubles and triples fire staff juggling with some fancy foot-work from Tim Marston.* Sep. 30, 2010.

4. *The Wind.* Jul. 3, 2009.

5. *Cinematique—Trailer.* Feb. 27, 2012.

6. *Isolation Hoop Report January '09.* Jan. 27, 2009.

7. *Rainbow's Birthday Teaser.* Jan. 21, 2010.

8. *Poi vs Isolation Hoops.* Mar. 8, 2009.

9. *Fan to Hoop Extravaganza!!!* Aug. 6, 2009.

10. *Le Cirque Éloize à l'émission "Des kiwis et des hommes."* Jul. 25, 2008.

11. *Laughing Yoga.* Dec. 31, 2008.

12. *AcroYoga Video Montage #2, AcroYoga Montreal 2010.* Jan. 1, 2010.

13. *Frenchy Hula Hooping at the NZJC.* Mar. 26, 2012.

14. *YogaSlackers Hanuman Slackline Hooping Fun.* Oct. 29, 2009.

15. *"Capoeira Angola from Salvador, Brazil" by Grupo de Capoeira Angola Pelourinho.* 1996.

16. *Lemonjelly Love.* Jul. 16, 2009.

17. *Zach and Marria NinjaHoops.* 2012.

18. *Hawaiian Dance.mp4.* Feb. 17, 2012.

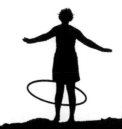

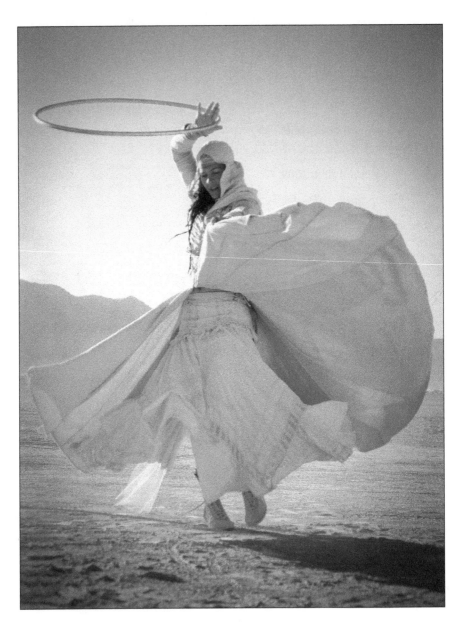

Spiral hoopdancing at Burning Man

ELEVEN

Spirit of the Hoop

The dancer's body is simply the luminous
manifestation of the soul.

—Isadora Duncan, visionary dancer

Mindfulness is the heart of hoopdance whether as a moving meditation, or for exercise that helps us improve self-awareness and sensory motor functions. Mindfulness practice handed down from the Buddhist tradition is used in Western psychology to facilitate mental, emotional, and physical wellness. In hoopdance, we bring complete attention to the present experience, learning without judgment. Right action, love, and creativity come about in surprising ways, over time, as we cultivate moment-to-moment consciousness.

The hoop is a static instrument of centrifugal force. Our moods and skill levels are ever changing. Bringing them together creates myriad opportunities to go beyond self. From American Indians and Christian fundamentalists to circus clowns and protesters, hoopdance promotes wellness and godliness through playfulness, personal growth, and compassionate service. Our thoughts and feelings focus on infinity as we twirl in a spirited blend of ecstatic dance, showmanship, and meditation. The Gnostic Gospel Acts of John 95 states: "Whoso danceth not, knoweth not what cometh to pass." Hoopdance is our window on the world. In its vortex our consciousness opens to divine suggestion, and the momentum of our goals increases.

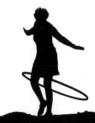

Prayer and Quest

Before Betty Shurin wrote the text of the Buddhist Heart Sutra on the surface of her early hoops, she had thought she was too self-conscious, rigid, and impatient to ever love dancing. Her sports were extreme and her thoughts and actions often obsessive or anxious. "In the hoop I forgot to worry, and the mindfulness that I experience in hoopdance changed the overall quality of my whole life. We can talk for years about what we want to release or manifest, but growth toward abundance actually *happens* when we awaken energy through intentional movement."

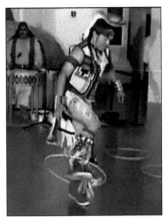

American Indians bring culture to life through their sacred storytelling hoop dances. As few as four hoops, and as many as thirty, invoke the essence of animals or themes in nature. Fanned out along the arms they become butterfly wings. Interlocking overhead they describe a three-dimensional sphere, echoing the earth orbiting in our solar system. Dancers embody the spirit of each design they create, moving with speed and grace to drumbeats and chanting. Derrick Davis, Hopi-Choctaw and four-time world champion hoop dancer, says, "There is medicine in our song, drumming, clothing, and dance. Hoop dancers are vehicles to share a message. When people watch, they are uplifted."[1] V

Tisha Marina uses the healing power of hoopdance as she travels around the country teaching nonviolence skills to stop bullying in schools. When she heard about the American Indian hoop dancer Sage Romero from her godparents, she wanted to meet him. "I wanted to learn about the sacred dances Sage performs with hoops and share my love of hooping with him." She thought it unlikely for this to happen because she is not Indian and Sage's dances are ceremonial in his culture. Then, when Tisha took over a class of middle-school students for two days, Sage turned out to be the class's regular teacher. He worked with Tisha, and they became friends.

Tisha had promised the students that if everyone listened throughout the nonviolence training, without talking over her words, she would show them some hoopdancing tricks. The students complied, and at the end of two productive days, they formed a circle around her in the yard, where she hooped for them. Then as a surprise, Sage came into the circle and performed as well. Tisha says, "We both had our own hoops and very different ways of using them. It was a rare experience for all. Like me, none of Sage's students had seen him dance. The children loved it." In *The Hooping Life* documentary, Tisha and other contemporary hoopdancers meet American Indian dancers, and they try each other's hoops.[2] [V]

Hooping in the Kingdom of the Light

Christian spirit grounds Dana Moore, the founder of AuraHoops. The first time she experienced an anointing of the Holy Spirit while dancing, she was in a stadium filled with candles at a Christian vigil. Music was playing, and the lyrics rang out: "Who am I that the Lord of all the earth would care to know my name? Little me. . . . " Dana started hoopdancing in a darkened corner of the field. "Something came over me. I had never been athletic or graceful, but I was twisting and whirling and flinging my hoop around like I never had before. At that 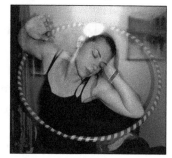 moment I left this earth and was in heaven. In my hoopdance, my heart and God's heart were totally connected. Bitterness has no choice but to flee when exposed to such light."

Dana had taken up hoopdance after a divorce that left her working two jobs. At her cocktail-waitress job a colleague noticed how irritable Dana was and said, "You had better pick up my hoop and work out your anger." Dana took that advice seriously, and every night after her children were in bed, she used her friend's water-filled toy hoop for hours. When she broke it, she added more water and taped it back together. It busted. She retaped it.

Believing she had been given the hoop for a reason, Dana asked, "Lord, what do You want me to do?" Then, using a concordance to the Bible, she looked up every instance of the word "dance" that is used in the text. She was struck by a definition for the word "chuwl," to twist or whirl in a

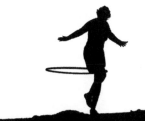

circular or spiral manner. "That's what I do when I hoop. Like David who slew Goliath in the Bible and was always dancing and whirling around."

Two years later Dana married her soulmate, Benjamin. She learned how to make a better hoop and started her Christ-centered dance and fitness company. "I use my gift grounded in God's Word. In return God blesses me with the fruits of the Spirit: kindness, gentleness, goodness, faith, love, long suffering, and peace." She overcomes her spiritual battles through hoopdance. The Holy Spirit inspires her movements and she responds without inhibition, as a form of prophetic dance, "interpreting His Word." [3] [V]

Dana and her family hosted us in Alabama when Nico Gerbi and I were on our month-long research trip by car. She served us a home-cooked breakfast the morning we got back on the road, and Nico fell in love with her fluffy Southern biscuits. After that we had to stop at Cracker Barrel every chance we got.

Walking for a Better World

Hoopdancer and clothing designer Ahni Radvanyi made her hoopdance quest on foot. Born Joanna Schulz, she gave herself a new name when she turned twenty-one. "'Ah,'" she says, "represents the primordial breath of all life, the exhalation that all humans share, and 'ni' echoes Radvanyi, which honors my matriarchal Hungarian family." Then, as an intern at Quail Springs Permaculture Farm in Ojai, California, Ahni studied living with integrity on the land that sustains us all. Inspired to encourage others in their own next steps toward a healthier environment, body, and consciousness, she embarked on a hoop hike.

During the summer of 2009 Ahni set out from Ojai and hooped continuously for 124 miles. On the road she carried her sleeping bag, a knife, a cell phone, and a GPS tracking system to record her mileage. For up to fifteen hours at a time, she hooped as she walked and danced through Ventura, Carpinteria, Goleta, Gaviota, ending her journey in Santa Barbara. "People I talked with all along the way got to see hooping as a metaphor for becoming the change within whichever circles they were dancing. Their smiling faces gave me encouragement."

As she was organizing her adventure, Ahni asked her friends and their friends for places to stay at night. Then she scheduled stops every fifteen to seventeen miles along the route. She was grateful for people who opened their homes to her so that she could take a shower and have a place to sleep. Some of them have become good friends. "Essentially I walked to one home and then another. On the nights I had no host, I slept in city parks with my hoop right next to me." Her adventure was written up in a *Santa Barbara News-Press* article.

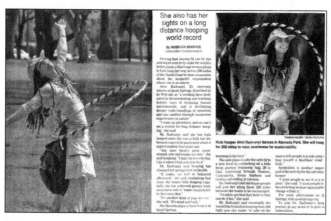

Connection and sharing were Ahni's favorite parts of the journey. Friends and other hoopers joined her along parts of the route. "A woman named Cricket hooped with me on the beach for part of a day, and my friend Victor played his guitar as we walked five or so miles near Rincon Beach. In another spot it felt like I had a little traveling circus going down the road, with Julian Gregg juggling as we walked along."

During most of the trip Ahni's feelings were of deep gratitude. "It was a beautiful kind of peaceful clarity, to wake up and know that my day was going to be as simple as walking and hooping. I watched the world go by, and each day became a meditation." She was uplifted when people recognized what she was doing. In Alta Vista, the community of street people seemed to know ahead of time that she was coming. One man called out when he saw her, "You're the girl who's hooping forever!" On the same corner someone else yelled back, "No, man, she's going five thousand miles." They had exaggerated, but nonetheless it was clear that her story had preceded her. Another man accompanied her to the house where she was staying that night. "It felt awesome that someone would take the initiative to walk with me for safety when it was getting dark."

At other times Ahni became exhausted. On a day after she had already walked about ten or twelve miles, she was disheartened at the prospect of a long and slow uphill climb for two or three more miles. "I was tired and the blisters on my feet were screaming. I couldn't make it up that hill. I collapsed into a stranger's yard. Unable to get up, I had to pee, which I did sitting right there on the lawn." Humiliated she began to cry. She was at the bottom of her own well. But before ten minutes had passed, a man came out of the house and wordlessly handed her a bottle of water. He had only smiled and gone back into the house, but his kindness worked like magic. "A drink from that bottle filled me with so much more than water. I was able to stand up, start spinning again, and continue. Moments like that remind me that even when we hit rock bottom, if only we are ready to receive it, there can be an invisible support system to help us get back up."

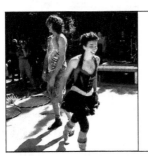

Ahni is also a street performer. She and Fabio are fabulous.[4] V

Personal Centering

Hoopdance combines the power of purposeful masculine strategy, stored in muscle memory, with uninhibited feminine movement, in a tangible symbol of unity—the circle of the hoop. Laura Blakeman's hooping name, Shakti Sunfire, embodies the union of feminine and masculine energies. The Hindu goddess Shakti personifies divine feminine vitality in polarity with the masculine Shiva. Shiva represents the essential elements of the universe that the potent Shakti brings to life.

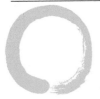

Pema Chödrön says in her Buddhist text *The Wisdom of No Escape* that by drawing a circle around ourselves we create a sacred space that becomes the center of the universe.

Shakti Sunfire follows the mantra "Begin Within." She lives her passion, leads with her heart, and pursues bliss for the good of all, embracing both strength and vulnerability. "If we start from inside to connect with universal consciousness, our energy ripples out to affect the greater community." She helps her students become comfortable in their bodies, urging us to reach out for hoop tosses. Teaching us to roll the hoop over our bodies from one outstretched arm to the other. Giving us permission to take up space. She prompts us to become twice our body height or width holding a hoop outstretched. "That can feel intimidating," she says, "but it also expands your size in the best possible way." [5] V

In school Laura had been a tomboy who wanted to be a cheerleader but couldn't do the splits. After college she started Kaivalya Hoopdancers with her friend Stephinity and established weekly public hoop jams at the Boulder Circus Center in Colorado. Hoopdance led Shakti Sunfire to aerial dance, which involves performing acrobatics, including the splits, on fabric that has been draped from the ceiling. "Hooping," she says, "burst open a whole world of optional ways for me to live that are completely in alignment with my values."

Beyond Oneness

When KaRa Maria Ananda came to California, Bunny Star and I were in her Hoop Mandala class at Hoopcamp. KaRa makes hoops with healing gems inside. She believes that hoopdance not only keeps the human body in good health but strengthens the Milky Way as well. "Much like the human heart," she explains, "our galaxy needs an energetic and steady pace for forming new stars and planets before growing old and quiet. As we spin our hoops, we are helping to regulate our galaxy's heartbeat as well as our own."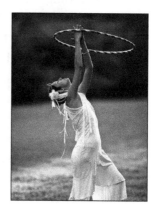

Bunny Star works in Sydney, Australia, teaching hoopdance in schools throughout the year and working on creative media projects during her

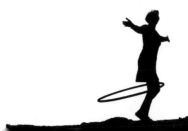

breaks. For regeneration and to deflect the burnout that can come from overwork or stress, she attends gatherings that connect her with her deepest source of vitality. At a Sacred Circularities retreat in Bali, Bunny improvised with a group of spiritually vibrant women in a natural healing environment. When she was introduced to Sufi whirling, she realized, "That motion is in my body as well."

Bunny is a devoted astrologer with a holographic view of life. She has studied the Bhagavad Gita and the teachings of Krishna, and is a bit of a Buddhist hybrid. She believes not only that hooping connects us with the spinning that is in all matter, including the planets and stars, but that we are all each other's spiritual masters. "We must defy prescribed spirituality a little bit to find God within," she says. "Refracted light causes human beings to mirror, illuminate, and interfere with each other. The person right in front of you is your teacher in that moment."

Before Julia Hartsell founded Hoop Convergence in North Carolina, she had read about the Sufis' whirling worship but didn't delve deeply into the poetic works of their leader, Jelaluddin Rumi, until she began hoopdancing. Rumi's followers founded the order of the Mevlevi, the whirling dervishes, and created the Sema, their sacred dance, as a mystical journey of spiritual ascent through mind and love to a state of perfection. Dervishes aim to be of service to the whole of creation without discriminating against beliefs, races, classes, and nations.

In college Julia was particularly drawn to the stories of mystical sects. She studied comparative religion, reading classical texts like *The Varieties of Religious Experience* by William James. Once she had earned her undergraduate degree, she trained in yoga and took belly-dance classes, longing for her own visceral spiritual awakening. Hoopdance set her on a path of meditation through movement. "The next thing you know," she says, "I had a religious experience like the ones I had read about."

It happened at the Carrboro Music Festival on Rumi's birthday. Julia was drawn to a room that had been used by the Rumi Fest during the day. Two bands were playing there in the evening, and the space was alive with a palpable energy when she started to hoopdance. As the music ended, she felt her heart open. She sat down, and with closed eyes, she saw a white light dancing with the hoop, ungrounded, out in the cosmos. "I felt the connection beyond oneness, without fear of death. I saw for myself the place I'm going to when I pass. Hooping is training me to return to the all, because everything is spinning."

Flow and Let Go

Hoopdance drills helped Khan Wong, producer of the Flow Show in San Francisco, to recognize his energetic connection with all life. After work-

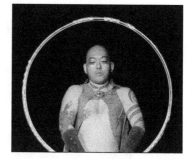

ing out a series of moves logically, he was breathing into them in repetition to make them flow more smoothly. "For the first time I felt a physical sensation of chi, the universal life force. It flowed through my body in sync with the patterns my hoop was creating. It felt as if time had stopped." He had experienced something similar with writing, when his words were flowing and he looked up to see that hours had passed, but this was a physical understanding and one he can't replicate at will. "You can't experience letting go by working at it. The experience of creative flow happens when it is unexpected."[6] [V]

As Khan became more known in the hoopdance community, friends urged him to perform and teach. Peer pressure compelled him to come up with new moves and to learn the more advanced tricks that were developed by other people. "I struggle to hold onto practice for the sake of practicing. The reward is simply to share the beauty of flow art whenever I can."

Inspired Service

Khan went on tour with the Laughing for Life Circus in 2008. Andrea Russell, a Canadian *poi* dancer living in Thailand, had gathered the group together. The circus show included spinning arts, acrobatic balancing, contact juggling, break dancing, and traditional Thai dance. Performers were from Ireland, Sweden, Spain, Bangkok, the island of Koh Samui, Holland, Japan, and the United States. Khan says, "We were spinning with fire in villages of huts with thatched roofs. It made me very nervous, but thankfully we didn't burn anything down."

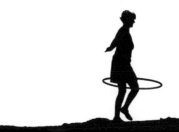

The audience included hill-tribes people, and Burmese refugees who cross the Moei River into Thailand when faced with starvation in their home country. The Thai Hmong and Akha Karen were in a situation somewhat like that of the American Indians in the late nineteenth and early twentieth centuries. They had no documentation in the form of deeds to property. Communities, culture, and livelihoods were threatened by men with guns who could drive families from land they had lived on for generations.

The group's shows and workshops were primarily for children. Many of them were Burmese orphans less than ten years old who had been liv-

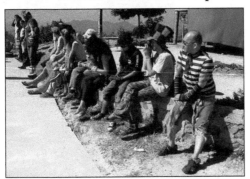

ing on the streets. Others had been rescued from the sex trade. Khan says, "The exuberance with which we were greeted was profoundly moving. The kids had harder lives than many of us could imagine, they are citizens of no country, yet they are filled with love." Faced with a language barrier, the troupe counted on Thai and Chinese translators a great deal, but teaching the children actually involved just a few words: "left," "right," "up," and "down" usually did the trick.

The Laughing for Life Circus was renamed Spark! Circus as it continued to grow. Andrea Russell says, " 'Spark' captures what we do as a volunteer fire circus, and it translates better into Thai." The Laughing for Life video from 2008 is six minutes of a-day-in-the-life style.[7] Ⓥ The one for Spark! Circus in 2010 is interview based.[8] Ⓥ

Cirques Ahoy

Performers who tour with a charitable circus share rooms, work hard, and sometimes see extreme poverty and violence. In 2004 Jo Wilding began bringing a collective of clowns to Iraq. Clowns hold a privileged place in most societies throughout the world, and they are often allowed to get away with breaking rules. In its first six years Circus 2 Iraq put on 270 shows, bringing laughter and hoops to over fifty thousand children. Since then the project has traveled to other regions of the Middle East, including

Palestine, Israel, Egypt, Jordan, and Kurdistan. Performers pay their own expenses for transportation and living, and raise funds by putting on events in the United Kingdom during the autumn months.

Sheila Hanney, representing the group, says, "In the course of our travels we donate funds directly to local enterprises that don't get money from the big charities. We put cash into the hands of small groups to help them clean up their environments or realize community projects." Efforts have included work on a sewage drainage system in an Iraqi refugee camp, sewing groups in the West Bank, and securing rehearsal space in Cairo where Egyptians collaborate with Iraqi refugees on theater projects.

Before setting off to the Middle East, performers train together at the Clown School in Bristol, England, where they get acquainted and cre-

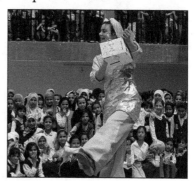

ate new shows. Then they take the loving silliness they develop directly to people who need it most: the children and families at risk because of war in the heart of the world. It's a serious mission in which playing games transcends barriers to physical and mental happiness. Founder Jo Wilding says, "Women are particularly important on our tours. As girls in the Middle East are given less freedom, it is more important to see women on the stage. A nine-foot-tall lady in a shiny frock makes them happy, and more girls will join group games when there are women to play with."

World Hoop Day

Many of us will never join the circus, but World Hoop Day gives us an opportunity to make a contribution through hoopdance. Annie Leffingwell O'Keeffe (Hoopin' Annie) founded World Hoop Day in New York, deciding that hoopdance was important enough to claim a holiday. In 2005 she spread the word everywhere she went and got her first media coverage in Vienna.[9] [V]

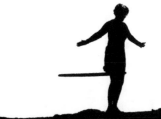

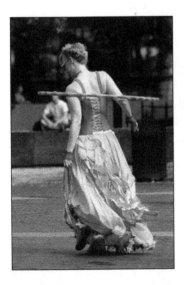

The first World Hoop Day (WHD) wasn't officially celebrated until July 7, 2007 (07-07-07). Then dates were set for 08-08-08, 09-09-09, and so on. To find dates after 12-12-12, check the website at www.WorldHoopDay.org. World Hoop Day presents a threefold mission:

- Get as many people as possible hooping for peace on the same day.

- Bring the joy of hooping into your own community first.

- Spread the culture of hoopdance wherever you travel in the world.

When Annie proposed the idea, people asked, "Why a holiday?" and "What's it for?" She countered, "Hoops are cheap to make, and hoopers are constantly giving them to each other, so how about giving hoops to the less advantaged wherever there is poverty, be it in Mexico or in New York City?" The idea caught on, and word traveled fast over the Internet. Philo Hagen featured World Hoop Day online at Hooping.org and interviewed Annie, which led others to contact her, asking what they could do to help or how they could sponsor an event in their town. Annie says, "I just pulled ideas out of the air and told them to make it grassroots. If you need a permit from your city, get one; if not, just gather together in a park. Make it simple."

In its first few years, Annie and Kevin O'Keeffe contributed $10,000 to fund the holiday. By 2009 more than fourteen thousand hoops valued at more than $83,000 had been given away to children and families at WHD events globally. In a village where Kevin had once lived near San Carlos, Mexico, he and Annie gave hoops to three schools and an orphanage that had no electricity; hoops were the perfect toy. When Annie travels, she teaches hooping to anyone who wants to learn—adult or child. Her personal goal is to spread peace and hooping as a registered nurse traveling the world.

World Hoop Day Ambassadors

Anyone participating in World Hoop Day is automatically an ambassador. One year Laura Scarborough, founder of HoopCircle and MagHoops in Austin, Texas, vacationed with her sister in Gili 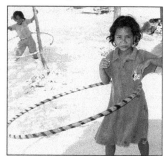 Trawangan, one of Indonesia's most remote islands. The island had no cars, police, or laws other than community tradition. When children saw Laura hooping on the beach, they sheepishly crept closer to watch. Laura says, "Of course we insisted they come and play. In no time at all they were laughing and encouraging one another." The evening before her departure, she gave all her hoops to the village. Later she received an e-mail telling her that the islanders held hooping contests. "The beautiful part is that hoops became a treasured possession not only for the kids but for the whole community. Sharing my love of hooping is one the of best things I do."

Gabriella Redding, CEO of Hoopnotica, went to Las Vegas from Los Angeles to lead a "hoop out" when the Las Vegas city council proposed a ban that threatened the 2010 WHD festivities. Gabriella publicly took issue with the city's intention to restrict hula hooping around the Fremont Street Experience, a seven-block open-air pedestrian mall featuring performance stages. If the ordinance had passed, street entertaining like hoopdance would be confined to established "free expression zones" abutting the mall. Gabriella protested: "The United States *is* a freedom of expression zone." A vote on the ban was successfully postponed as a result of the protest.[10] [V]

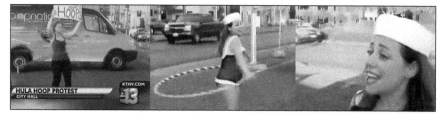

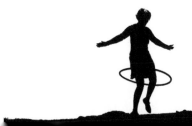

Julie Schoolastra helped Kaya Esperanza Somers organize the World Hoop Day event in Las Vegas that year. Julie had moved to Vegas from Southern California in 2008 and volunteered at a local food bank called Three Squares before helping to expand the hooping community and getting involved with WHD. Kaya founded Luv2Hoop and organized her first Vegas WHD celebration in 2008, after seeing Karis perform in a club.

Kaya had grown up poor in El Paso, Texas, but loved hula hooping as a kid. "I hoop; therefore I am. My mother made sacrifices for me and my sisters, and I want to make a difference in the lives of children in Clark County by sharing hoops." She and Julie made two hundred hoops for students attending the Fremont Middle School in Las Vegas's Clark County, the fifth largest school district in the country. The county donated the use of its Winchester Community Center. Money and in-kind donations came from individuals and local businesses. When families arrived at the community center, volunteers gave each child a hoop. There was music on the grassy lawn, with face painting, raffle prizes, and roaming hoop performances. Julie says, "The greatest thing about World Hoop Day is that adults and children play together. That helps build community."

Random Acts of Hooping

In 2005, Caroleeena established an annual hoop donation project in

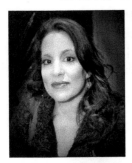

Negril, Jamaica, to give hoops to children who had never seen them before. Because there is no PVC pipe on the island and plumbing fittings are made of metal, Caroleeena and her friends take tubing, tape, and connectors with them to make the hoops they leave behind. In the fourth year of the project they visited a school library that had only fourteen books for 2,200 students. Caroleeena says, "We kicked up our efforts and donated eighty-eight books and sixty-six backpacks, plus art supplies."

That was the year she met Fred Tackett, a founding member of the Little Feat Band. The band's annual fans' retreat was held at one of Jamaica's luxury resorts. "I asked Fred if his guests, who were much more wealthy than our crew, would bring two books each as well as a musical instrument to place with a student or a school." It was a huge success.

In North Carolina, Caroleeena mobilized a World Hoop Day drive to craft and give away forty-four hoops to pediatric AIDS patients through Duke University Hospital. Earlier that summer she hosted a hoop jam for the Governor Morehead School for the Blind. "I believe that anything we love to do can be done as a service, and our service to others is also a gift to ourselves. Helping you helps me. Imagine what the world would be like if more people understood that."

Chance Encounter

In Berkeley I received a spontaneous teaching on a day when I was sharing hoops in the park. I had started the music player and begun to hoopdance when a woman I had never seen before approached. "Such movement," she exclaimed. "It is the movement of women!" Her heart-shaped face beamed with pleasure. Her feet were bare, but her stride was solid and strong, and the modestly fitted dress she wore was perfect for hooping. Her name was Suriya, and she asked if the two preteen neighborhood girls who had climbed into a nearby tree might use my extra hoops. "Yes, of course," I said, "and you should too."

I wasn't sure what the relationship was between Suriya and the girls, but they clearly trusted her. They scrambled down and got right into hooping. They had done it before. Suriya hadn't. I showed her the basic movement, and she soon had a large hoop successfully spinning. As I taught the girls various ways to manipulate their hoops, our exchanges were lively and loud. Unexpectedly, Suriya stopped me and suggested that I stop smiling, chewing gum, and using words. That gave me pause. The night before I had been in my kitchen, standing on one leg to test my coordination for one-legged hooping. I was less steady than I had been when I practiced this as a yoga stance in my youth, and I wondered if I needed a teacher. Now Suriya was here instructing me.

I threw my gum into a nearby trash container and returned to her quietly, with relaxed facial muscles.

"Squeeze my hand very tightly," she said, and I did.

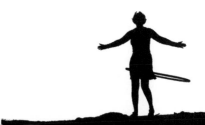

When I resumed hooping, she told me to drop my personality, which is largely made up of smiles, and she stood watch. "Close your eyes," she said. "Move the water in you, not your bones and muscles.

"Feel the energy in your core.

"Stop using your body.

"Shift your weight.

"Don't be symmetrical."

I thanked her for giving me a new way to practice.

"Don't practice," she admonished. "You need to be like cold water. Does the mountain spring practice getting to the sea? No. It just falls fearlessly!"

I stayed with Suriya in the park for hours. She lifted me in her arms as I reached to the sky, and she set me down to sink to the earth. I hooped in one direction and then the other, stretching my fingers away from upturned palms, eyes closed, and barely moving. She sang and breathed out strong guttural sounds to accompany my blindness, stopping to tell me that I was smiling or that I was flowing like water. Then we sat on the grass, and she said that I had visited her as a spirit the previous evening, and that because I was born in 1946 and was sixty-four years old, I was entering the spiritual quarter of my life. She said, "The hoop is a tool. You don't need it."

I haven't seen Suriya again, but her teaching stays with me as I deepen my hoopdance practice. She inspired me in many ways; some things she said I may not fully understand for years to come, but daily I practice dropping my personality by quieting my thoughts and restraining my smiles, continuing my hoopdance practice with an internal focus.

Chapter Eleven Links

www.HoopDanceBook.com/chapter11

1. *Amazing Indian Hoop Dance.* May 20, 2007.
2. *The hoopers explore their roots—The Hooping Life Film.* Sep. 16, 2009.
3. *WaitForMe.* Jun. 29, 2009.
4. *"Hit Snap Clap Hoopla!" with AHni and Fabio.* Jun. 9, 2010.
5. *Shakti Sunfire in Flow.* Nov. 6, 2011.
6. *Flow Show 2: Unlock.* Apr. 19, 2010.
7. *Laughing For Life 2008 part 1.* Apr. 20, 2008.
8. *Spark! Circus 2010 Tour.* Sep. 13, 2010.
9. *World Hoop Day's First Media Hit.* May 30, 2007.
10. *Las Vegas Hula Hoop Protest: 10.* Sep. 8, 2010.

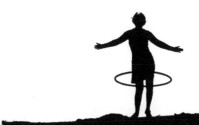

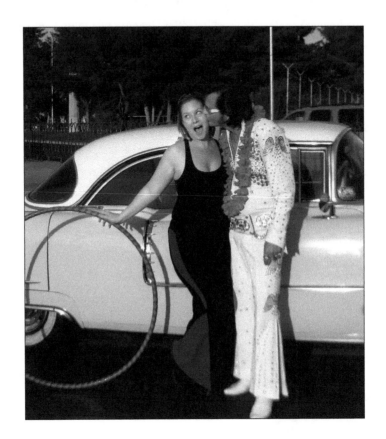

Julie Schoolastra with Elvis impersonator

Acknowledgments

Writing this book took a village of many more friends and contributors than is possible to mention in its pages. Deep gratitude goes to everyone who lent their stories and images, to Cay Lang for uttering the idea that I would write a book about hoopdance, to Joell Jones for setting an example, to Andrea and Wes McLean for wardrobe and lifelong encouragement, and especially to Tom Weidlinger for providing the unflinching editorial and video support that helped to make the book readable and visual.

Special thanks to Paula Morrison, Gretchen Lemke-Santangelo, and Shailja Patel for believing and guiding, to Nico Gerbi for research assistance, and to Andrew Kaluzinski for help with the book's video trailer.

Thank you Christine Ravish for starting the story, and Kaye Anderson for illustrating moves in the studio.

Thanks to Carolyn North, Jeanne Jabbour, Jan Freeman Long, Sass Colby, Peri Fletcher, Mick Renner, Nadia Kameli, James Cline, Dick Stein, Marcy Voyevod, Sophie Elliott, Sterling Gee, Ayelet Maida, and Marsha Thomas Cooke for comments and enthusiasm; to Ginger Theisen, Laura Daughtery, Renee Kogler, Adam Parsons, Julie Siegel, Dana Moore, Nadia Sophia, Julia Harsell, Lewis Dolinsky, Zeph Chmura, and Blake Jones for hospitality; to Hanna Chauvet for technical support; and to Beth Wright and Zan Ceeley for copy editing and proofing.

Finally, thanks to Zach Fischer and Marria Grace for hooping at Marin Headlands for the cover of the book; and to everyone else who shared their photos inside.

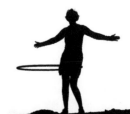

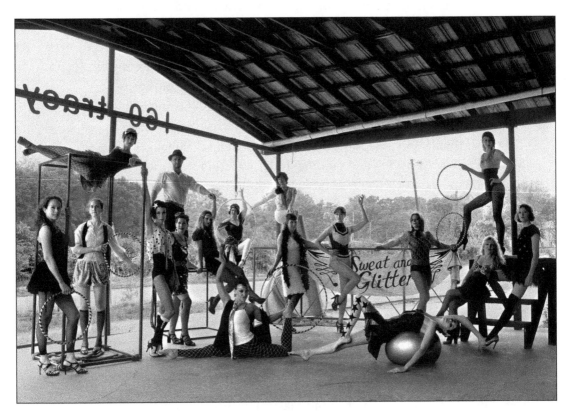

Canopy Studio Repertory Theater

Revolutionary Resources

Check the website for updates.

Photographers

Neil Anderson. www.cameranotesneilandersen.com
   Photo of tandem hoopdancing, page 156.

Joey Cardella, JoeySee. www.joeysee.com
   Photo of Spiral, page 210.

Sally Cox, Happy Hula Monkeys. www.hoopshaker.com
   Photo of Julie with Elvis impersonator, page 228.

C. Taylor Crothers. www.ctaylorcrothers.com
   Photo of String Cheese Incident, courtesy of Madison House
   Publicity, 2005, page 99.

John Dart, John Dart Photography. www.johndartphotography.com
   Photo of KC Mendicino, page 116.

Terry Lee Dill. www.terryleedill.com
   Photo of BunnyMan, page 19.

Brandy Engles. www.brandyengle.tumblr.com
   Photo of Caroleeena, page 37.

Tony Fototaker. www.fototaker.net
   Photo of Isa Isaacs, page 170.

Matt Freedman. www.facebook.com/MattFreedmanPhotography
   Photo of Spiral, page xiv.

Ben Fullerton. www.fullertonimages.com
   Photo of Adelaide and Sam, page 204.

April Garzarek, CaptureStudios. www.facebook.com/CaptureStudios
   Photo of Carolyn Mabry, page 224.

Austin Green. www.facebook.com/austin.green.fierce
   Photo of Brandy Hughes, page 91.

Laurie Hobbs. Threshold Photography www.facebook.com/zemaya
   Photo of Beth Lavinder, page 45.

Barry J. Holmes. www.barryjholmes.com
   Photo of Rich and Spiral, page 193.

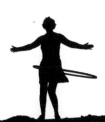

Jasper Johal. www.jasperphoto.com
  Photo of Adelaide and Sam, page 191.

Cay Lang. www.caylang.com
  Photos of Kaye Anderson, pages 29–32 (illustrations), page 201.

Taymar LaRue. www.facebook.com/taymar
  Photos of Revolva, pages 148 and 161.

Jessica Lobdell, Jessica Lobdell Photography. www.jessicalobdell.com
  Photo of Scott and Julia Crews, page 183.

Brandon Miller. www.johnbrandonmiller.com
  Photos of the Seattle fashion show, page 170.

Justin Monroe. www.justinmonroe.com
  Photo of Mr. Dead poster, page 154.

Scott Patrick, Scott Patrick Photography. www.scottpatrick.com
  Photos of Stephanie Babines, page 85.

Shane Riggs. www.facebook.com/roryshaneinmd
  Photo of Aaron Smith, page 94.

Marta Sasinowska. www.flickr.com/photos/mart_ai
  Photo of Grant's wedding at Burning Man, page 180.

Louis M. Seigal. www.seigalphotography.com
  Photo of Annie O'Keeffe, page 222.

Ralph Singer. www.2ralph.com
  Photo of whirling dervishes, page 39.

Sean Stuchen. www.seanstuchen.com
  Photo of KaRa Maria Ananda, page 217.

Steve Wilson.
  Photo of Nadia Sophia, page 206.

Kyer Wiltshire. www.kyerwiltshire.com
  Photo of Spiral, page 112.

Pilar Woodman. www.pilarwoodmanphoto.com
  Photo of Heather Toles, page 67.

Hoopdancers

KaRa Maria Ananda, Hoop Alchemy
  www.hoopalchemy.com
  www.facebook.com/karaananda

Kaye Anderson, Hoop Power
  www.hoop-power.com
  www.facebook.com/kayelcsw

Stephanie Babines, Oh My You're Gorgeous
www.OhMyYouReGorgeous.com

Steve Bags (Bags)
www.facebook.com/steve.bags.5
www.youtube.com/steve2bags

Jonathan Livingston Baxter (Baxter), HoopPath
www.hooppath.com
www.facebook.com/jonathan.baxter
www.youtube.com/user/jlbaxter

Paul Blair (Dizzy Hips)
www.dizzyhips.net
www.facebook.com/dizzyhoops
www.youtube.com/user/DizzyHips

Laura Blakeman (Shakti Sunfire)
www.shaktisunfire.com
www.facebook.com/shaktisunfire

Nayeli Michelle Bouvier, HoopNectar
www.hoopnectar.com
www.facebook.com/nayelishakti
www.youtube.com/user/HoopNectar

Faerie Cara, Eco Faeries
www.ecofaeries.com
www.facebook.com/ecofaeries
http://www.youtube.com/user/ecofaeries

Michele Clark
www.facebook.com/oracledance
www.youtube.com/user/spin0da0rella

Jon Coyne, Hoopsmiles
www.facebook.com/jonpcoyne
www.youtube.com/user/hoopsmiles

Patrick Deluz, PsiHoops
www.psihoops.com
www.youtube.com/user/PsiHoops

Kacey Douglas (Miss Hoopstress), Homespun Hoops
www.homespunhoops.com
www.facebook.com/homespun.hoops

Lara Eastburn, Superhooper
www.superhooper.org
www.facebook.com/lara.eastburn

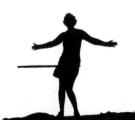

Zach Fischer, Ninja Hoops
www.ninjahoops.com
www.facebook.com/zfischer1
www.youtube.com/user/NinjaHoops

Claire French (Frenchy), Frenchy Productions
www.frenchyproductions.com

Josette Gasse
www.facebook.com/elmagasse

Gems Goddard
www.facebook.com/hoopgems
www.youtube.com/user/gemmyuk

Jocelyn Gordon, HoopYogini
www.jocelyngordon.com
www.facebook.com/JocelynGordon.lovemovement

Marria Grace, Ninja Hoops
www.ninjahoops.com
www.facebook.com/marriagrace
www.youtube.com/user/NinjaHoops

Nick Guzzardo
www.facebook.com/nicguzz
www.youtube.com/user/nicnox

Vivian Hancock (Spiral), Hoop Technique
www.spiralhoopdance.com
www.spiralcircusarts.com
www.facebook.com/vivianspiral

Philo Hagen, Hooping.org
www.hooping.org
www.facebook.com/philohagen
www.youtube.com/user/philohagen

Julia Hartsell (Jewels)
www.hoopdrum.com
www.facebook.com/SpinningJewels
www.youtube.com/user/julahoop

Brandy Hughes (BHoops)
www.facebook.com/brandyhappyhug

Colleen Hurley, Twistin Vixens
www.twistinvixens.com
www.facebook.com/tvhooping
www.youtube.com/user/TwistinVixens

Bill Huson
  www.youtube.com/spinyang
  www.facebook.com/whuson

Kari Jones (Revolva)
  www.revolvahoopdance.com
  www.facebook.com/revolva
  www.youtube.com/user/revolva76

Emma Kerr, Hooping Mad
  www.hoopingmad.co.uk
  www.facebook.com/hoopingmad
  www.youtube.com/hoopingmad

Lynn Knickrehm-Fisher, Boisehoopla
  www.boisehoopla.com
  www.facebook.com/lynn.knickrehmfisher

Renee Kogler, Cleveland Hoopdance
  www.facebook.com/renee.kogler

Kayla Kuhlmann, Twistin Vixens
  www.twistinvixens.com
  www.facebook.com/tvhooping
  www.youtube.com/user/TwistinVixens

Beth Lavinder
  www.facebook.com/beth.lavinder
  www.youtube.com/user/lavinder5

Grant Leonard, Tropo
  www.facebook.com/grant.leonard

Rosie Lila (Miss Rosie)
  www.herohoops.com
  www.facebook.com/RosieLila

Diana Lopez, Body Hoops
  www.bodyhoops.com
  www.facebook.com/diana.lopez.hulahooper

Lisa Lottie
  www.lisalottie.com
  www.facebook.com/lisaxlottie
  www.youtube.com/user/lisaxlottie

Betty Lucas, Lucas Hooping
  www.lucashoopping.com
  www.facebook.com/LucasHooping

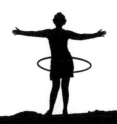

Carolyn Mabry (Caroleeena)
www.circlesofjoy.org
www.facebook.com/Caroleeena
www.youtube.com/user/Caroleeena

Bonnie MacDougall
www.havenhoopdance.com
www.facebook.com/havehoopdance

Van Maffei (Von), Hella Hoops
www.facebook.com/pages/Hella-Hoops/272850759468

Adelaide Marcus, Shimmy Sisters
www.artbyadelaide.com

Laura Marie, Hooping Harmony
www.hoopingharmony.com
www.facebook.com/pages/Hooping-Harmony/210252261853
http://www.youtube.com/user/hoopingharmony

Tisha Marina
www.facebook.com/TishaMarinaBernard

Jaguar Mary (Ja Má)
www.facebook.com/jaguarmaryx
www.youtube.com/user/jaguarmaryone

Rayna McInturf (Hoopnotica)
www.hooprevolution.com
www.facebook.com/rayna.mcinturf
www.youtube.com/user/raynamcinturf

Rainbow Michael
www.facebook.com/RainbowMichael

Jo Mondy, Live Love Hoop
www.livelovehoop.com www.facebook.com/jomondy
www.youtube.com/user/livelovehoop

Dana Moore, AuraHoops
www.facebook.com/groups/aurahoops

Gail O'Brien, Hoop Spin
www.hoopspin.co.uk
www.facebook.com/hoopspin
www.youtube.com/user/HoopSpin1

Annie O'Keeffe, World Hoop Day
www.worldhoopday.org
www.facebook.com/WorldHoopDay

Alley 'Oop
  www.alleyoophoop.com
  www.facebook.com/alley.oop.773
  www.youtube.com/user/AlleyOophoop

Stefan Pildes, Groovehoops
  www.groovehoops.com
  www.facebook.com/Groovehoops
  www.youtube.com/user/Groovehoops

Melanie Pleasure
  www.melaniepleasure.me
  www.facebook.com/pleasehoop

Mat Plendl
  www.matplendl.com
  www.facebook.com/mat.plendl
  www.youtube.com/user/matplendl

Rich Porter, Isopop
  www.isopop.com
  www.facebook.com/isopop
  www.youtube.com/user/r1chinSLO

Mona Qaddoumi, ShpongledHoops
  www.facebook.com/pages/Mona-ShpongledHoops/109756822380710
  www.youtube.com/user/shpongledhoops

Ahni Radvanyi
  www.etsy.com/shop/ahniradvanyi
  www.facebook.com/ahni.radvanyi
  www.youtube.com/user/ahniradvanyi

Gabriella Redding, Hoopnotica CEO
  www.hoopnotica.com
  www.facebook.com/gabriella.redding.3

Anah Reichenbach (Hoopalicious)
  www.hooprevolution.com
  www.facebook.com/hoopalicious

Fran Reichenbach (Mamalicious)
  www.facebook.com/fran.reichenbach

Brecken Rivara
  www.facebook.com/brecken.rivara

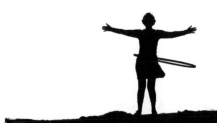

Sharna Rose
www.sharnarose.co.uk
www.facebook.com/sharna.bevan
www.youtube.com/user/sharnarose

Laura Scarborough, HoopCircle
www.hoopcircle.com
www.facebook.com/misslaurahere

Julie Schoolastra, Hooptopia
www.hooptopia.com
www.facebook.com/julie.schoolastra.5

Sandi Schultz (Sass)
www.cybersass.com
www.facebook.com/cybersass
www.youtube.com/user/cybersass

Ariana Shelton, Hooping Harmony
www.hoopingharmony.com
www.facebook.com/pages/Hooping-Harmony/210252261853
http://www.youtube.com/user/hoopingharmony

Betty Shurin (Betty Hoops)
www.bettyhoops.com
www.facebook.com/betty.hoops
www.youtube.com/user/bettyhooping

Megan Simpson, Hooper Troopers
www.hooper-troopers.com
www.facebook.com/megan.simpson

Dana Skelton, Athens Hoopdance
www.athenshoopdance.wordpress.com
www.facebook.com/danaskelton

Aaron Smith, Concentric Fire
www.facebook.com/aaron.smith.581730
www.youtube.com/user/smithaar12

Nadia Sophia
www.nadiasophia.com
www.facebook.com/nadiaxsophia
www.youtube.com/user/nadiasophia1

Bunny Star (Bunny Hoop Star)
www.hoopempire.com
www.facebook.com/bunnyhoopstar

Malcolm Stuart
  www.malcolmstuart.com
  www.facebook.com/malcolm.stuart.18
  www.youtube.com/user/malcolmstuart

Sandra Summerville (SaFire), HoopCity.ca
  www.hoopcity.ca
  www.sfiredance.com
  www.youtube.com/user/FireSandra

Heather Toles
  www.facebook.com/heather.toles.7

Heather Troy
  www.facebook.com/heather.troy.98

Karis Wilde (Karis)
  www.facebook.com/kariskaris

Khan Wong, SF Flow Show
  www.fundtheflowarts.org
  www.facebook.com/mutant.song
  www.youtube.com/user/mutantsong

Nicole Wong, Cherry Hoops
  www.cherryhoops.com
  www.facebook.com/CherryHoops

Natasha Young, Hoopsie Daisy
  www.hoopsiedaisy.com
  www.facebook.com/hoopsiedaisy

Christabel Zamor (HoopGirl)
  www.hoopgirl.com
  www.facebook.com/HoopGirl

International Retreats

Burning Man
  www.burning

Harbin Hoop Jam (Flowjam)
  www.melaniepleasure.me/hoopbliss

Hoopcamp
  www.hoopcampretreats.com

Hoop Convergence
  www.hoopconvergence.org

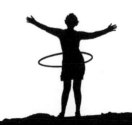

HoopPath
www.hooppath.com

Manchester Hoop Congress
www.hoopspin.co.uk/manchester-hoop-congress

Movement Play Microfestival
www.movementplay.com

SWHoop (South West Hoop Conference)
www.swhoop.co.uk

Sacred Circularities
www.sacredcircularities.com

Spin Matsuri
www.spinmatsuri.com

Spin Summit
www.thespinsummit.com

U.K. Hoop Gathering
www.ukhoopgathering.com

Hoops and Clothing

Hoops

Canyon Hoops by Ron Klint
www.canyonhoops.com

Discount Hoop Supplies by Sunny Becks-Crumpton
www.hoopsupplies.com

EcoHoop
www.hooprevolution.com

Infinity Travel hoop
www.bodyhoops.com
www.facebook.com/diana.lopez.hulahooper

Mag hoops
www.facebook.com/MagHoops
www.youtube.com/user/scarbiedoll

LED hoops
www.psihoops.com
www.youtube.com/user/PsiHoops

Polypro hoops
www.superhooper.org
www.superhooper.org/polyprovideoseries.html

Fire hoops
www.synergyflowarts.com
www.youtube.com/user/synergyfirehoops

Your Hoop by Jesica Flowers
www.yourhoop.com

Tape

www.Identi-Tape.com

Clothing

Alienskin by Kate Technodolly
www.alienskin.co.uk

Annieland by Annie Weinert
www.annieland.net

Mended Mosaic by KC Medicino
www.MendedMosaic.com

Onyx by Lauren Porter
www.onyxscloset.com

Music, Books, and DVDs

Music

DJ Spin Sisters with Sophia Mavrides.
www.djspinsisters.com
www.facebook.com/pages/Spin-Sisters/277916283466

Hoopdrum, Scott Crews
www.hoopdrum.com
www.facebook.com/scottwcrews
www.youtube.com/user/scottwcrews

"How to Hoop" rap song, Hoopsmiles (Jon Coyne)
www.youtube.com/user/hoopsmiles/store

The String Cheese Incident
www.stringcheeseincident.com

Tropo
www.reverbnation.com/tropo

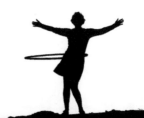

Books

Judith Lanigan. *The Hula Hoop: The First Compendium or Serious Study of the Subject,* Second Edition. Lulu.com. 2008 www.lulu.com/shop/product-3191420.html

Christabel Zamor with Ariane Conrad. *Hooping: A Revolutionary Fitness Program.* Workman Publishing Company. Inc., New York, NY, 2009. www.hoopgirl.com

eBooks

HoopGirl. www.hoopgirl.com
Minihoops eBook (all levels)

Hoopnotica. www.hoopnotica.com
Hooping Through Pregnancy

Tim Marston. www.howtosellyouract.com
How to Sell Your Act

DVDs

Betty Hoops. www.bettyhoops.com
HoopCore Fitness
4 Rhythm Hoop Dance
Kids Hoop Warrior

Bodyhoops. www.bodyhoops.com
Hoop Dance Fusion

Bunny Hoop Star. www.hoopempire.com
Hooping for Beginners

HoopGirl. www.hoopgirl.com
HoopDance For Beginners
Hoopdance Evolution (intermediate)
The Hoop Dance Workout (fitness)
Hulaerobics (beginner)

Hoopnotica. www.hoopnotica.com
Hoopdance Hula Hoop DVD Level 1 (Beginner)
Hoopdance Hula Hoop DVD Level 2 (Beginner)
Hoopdance Hula Hoop DVD Level 3 (Intermediate)
Hoopdance Hula Hoop DVD Level 4 (Intermediate)
Hula Hoop Minis DVD Level 1

Hoop Path. www.hooppath.com
First Steps (beginner / inspirational)